WHAT TO
eat WHEN YOU'RE pregnant

WHAT TO
eat
WHEN YOU'RE
pregnant

A week-by-week
GUIDE TO SUPPORT
YOUR HEALTH AND YOUR
BABY'S DEVELOPMENT

NICOLE M. AVENA, PhD
Recipes by Georgie Fear, RD

TEN SPEED PRESS
Berkeley

Published in the United States by Ten Speed Press,
an imprint of the Crown Publishing Group, a division
of Penguin Random House LLC, New York.
www.crownpublishing.com
www.tenspeed.com

Ten Speed Press and the Ten Speed Press colophon are registered
trademarks of Penguin Random House, LLC.

Avena, Nicole M., 1978–
What to eat when you're pregnant : a week-by-week guide to support your
health and your baby's development / Nicole M. Avena, PhD; recipes by Georgie Fear, RD.
        pages cm
Summary: "A week-by-week guide to what to eat—as opposed to what to avoid—while
pregnant and nursing, to support the mother's health and the baby's development during
each stage of pregnancy, with 50 recipes"—Provided by publisher.
Includes bibliographical references and index.
1. Pregnancy—Nutritional aspects. 2. Mothers—Nutrition. 3. Fetus—Nutrition.
4. Cooking. I. Fear, Georgie. II. Title.
RG559.A94 2015
618.2—dc23
                    2015005472

Trade Paperback ISBN 978-1-60774-679-9
eBook ISBN 978-1-60774-680-5

Printed in the United States of America

Design by Kara Plikaitis

10 9 8 7 6 5 4 3 2 1

First Edition

Dedication

To Stella's sister.

Contents

Acknowledgments

I would especially like to acknowledge Regina Vaicekonyte, MS, who assisted with research on several elements of this book. Her expertise in nutrition was invaluable to this project. She was there at every step along the way, and her interest, ideas, and enthusiasm were all very much appreciated.

There are many additional important people to acknowledge and thank for their role in the development of this book.

Gratitude to Georgie Fear, RD, who developed the delicious and easy-to-prepare recipes, along with other key nutritional excerpts throughout the book. Her ideas for simple, practical meals are perfect for busy moms!

Thanks to Susan Murray for her keen eye, flair for writing, and devoted efforts assisting with the research, organization, editing, and pretty much anything and everything else needed for this book.

Thanks to my editor, Julie Bennett, and the entire team at Ten Speed Press as well as the Crown Publishing Group and Penguin Random House for their assistance and support. Working with you all has been a great experience—even more so the second time around!

Thanks to Alastair Tulloch, MS, for his input, research, and willingness to read through the manuscript as an "outsider" (although he is certainly not one!).

Thanks to Katie Bishop, MS, for her assistance researching parts of the book, even up until the last minute.

Thanks to Linda Konner for her sage advice and support throughout the development of this book and beyond.

Thanks to all of my colleagues and collaborators for their research and the valuable information they have produced in the fields of nutrition and developmental psychology. Not only has this information kept me fascinated by this topic, but it has also led to many interesting and educational discussions over the years.

I also thank my dear friends and family for their help and support along the way.

Gratitude to Deb Gutter and Stephanie Madeline, who took the time to give me detailed, helpful comments on the initial plan for this book.

Thanks to all of my mommy friends, who have allowed me to draw on their experiences during and after each of their unique pregnancies. MaryLynn Bohlayer, Nicole Sette, Beth Tengowski, Casey McElligott, Tara Todd, and Stas Weinstock have all been great friends and resources on many life matters, not just those related to babies.

I also owe an infinite amount of thanks to my husband, Eamon, whose support and encouragement keeps me going. Bert, thanks for reminding me to relax.

And last but not least, thanks to my darling baby, Stella, for inspiring me to write this book. We are blessed to have such a happy and healthy little girl, and I wish for every mom out there to be as fortunate. The journey of having you has been the most exciting experience I could have ever imagined, and every day it keeps getting better.

PART I

Why Is It Important to Eat Well during Pregnancy?

CHAPTER 1

Evolution of the Baby Bump and Being Pregnant Today

Congratulations! If you're reading this book, you are most likely at the beginning stages of a beautiful journey through pregnancy—or else thinking about embarking on it soon. Pregnancy can be a joyful life event; it is often celebrated with baby showers, pampering, and even "babymoons" (when a couple goes on vacation or a weekend getaway before the birth). Pregnancy is also a rite of passage. During and after pregnancy, women experience major physical, social, and psychological transitions, and their roles and responsibilities as individuals change dramatically and forever.

While pregnancy can be exciting and nerve-racking at the same time, it is also one of the most profound periods in a woman's life. You're sure to have many questions and concerns, especially if this is your first baby. *How do I ensure that my baby is healthy? What can I eat and what should I avoid while I'm pregnant? Will my body ever look the same after this? Will I be a good mom?* If you are anything like I was when I got pregnant with my daughter, you are probably also feeling sheer excitement and happiness intermixed with these worries.

Let Food Be Thy Medicine

The primary concern of every pregnant woman is the health and well-being of her growing baby, and science suggests that what we eat while pregnant can have dramatic effects on the baby's development and behavior later in life.

But trying to eat healthy is hard in the modern food environment, especially when you are pregnant. Also, what does "eating healthy" even mean anymore? There is so much conflicting information out there about what to eat, it can make your head spin.

In addition to doing research in this field, I also have firsthand experience with the trials and tribulations of eating well during pregnancy and beyond. When I first became pregnant with my daughter, I was overwhelmed with excitement. I started to read every book and web article I could find about pregnancy. That's when the fear began to set in. It seemed like *everything* was potentially toxic or damaging to a growing baby. Between avoiding kitty litter and wondering if the cheese I'd bought was pasteurized, I wanted to hide in my house or surround myself with BPA-free bubble wrap for the next nine months. Plus, I quickly began to realize that following weight-gain guidelines was easier said than done.

As a neuroscientist with a focus on appetite and nutrition, I spend most of my days thinking about and testing how what we eat affects our brains. I know that the foods we eat can dramatically affect our behavior and health, and this is even more critical when it comes to the nourishment that a pregnant woman passes along to her developing baby. However, as a pregnant woman I found the information out there for me and other moms-to-be confusing, limited, and overwhelmingly focused on the negatives: avoid this, avoid that. I found myself wondering, *After we avoid all of those foods, what should we eat?* I am also a skeptical person by nature (probably fueled by my training to become a scientist), and I wanted to know not just *what* to eat, but also *why*, and I wanted some proof to back it up. I wasn't sold on the old wives' tales.

I wanted to write this book to help mothers-to-be better understand what they should eat when expecting, and why. In addition to avoiding the bad things, we can capitalize on the good things that foods can do to promote health at critical points during development. Also, I know that eating well can be a challenge, especially when so much of today's commercial food offerings are junk. This challenge can become even greater when compounded by the social norms surrounding pregnancy and the hormones and mood changes that occur over those nine-plus months.

The goal of this book is to sift through the rumors and media stories to give you a real account of the science behind why your weight and what you eat during pregnancy are important for you and your baby, as well as to provide you with a practical plan of what to eat for the best outcome. Not only will eating the foods described in the following chapters help you keep your weight in check during and after pregnancy, but also by eating foods that are rich in key nutrients at critical points throughout your pregnancy, you will help your baby grow up strong and healthy.

The Evolution of Pregnancy Myths and Reality

Over the centuries, people have viewed pregnancy in ways that may seem not only foreign but also a bit crazy. For example, in the first and second century it was believed that your thoughts during pregnancy could affect your offspring—all because one Greek physician noted that pregnant women who thought about monkeys delivered hairy children! Similarly, in the eighteenth century, it was thought that the incidence of birth defects, such as babies being born deaf or blind, resulted directly from mothers' experiences while expecting, such as having been shocked by a loud sound or having looked at a blind person. Pregnancy was not always managed by doctors; in fact, for most of human history, information was passed down from mother to daughter or conveyed by (often untrained) midwives. Expectant women were traditionally told all sorts of old wives' tales, myths, and ancient wisdom (which, in hindsight, wasn't always so wise!) about the secrets to a healthy pregnancy and newborn.

Over the last hundred years, however, pregnancy has become highly medicalized. It has also become an area of intense scientific research, with more findings now than ever before. The research exploring how maternal behavior during pregnancy may impact a child's health and development has helped us move beyond folk tales and get to the facts about what expectant mothers should or shouldn't do during pregnancy to promote optimal health for both their babies and themselves.

It Starts with Food

One of the first inklings of the importance of prenatal nutrition came from the consequences of a natural phenomenon known as the Dutch winter famine. During the winter and spring of 1944, the German army rationed the food supply in parts of the Netherlands. It was later found that women who were pregnant during this time were more likely to have had children with various health problems, including being either too small or obese and having greater rates of cardiovascular disease. These findings sparked a slew of research on the impact of maternal undernutrition, such as protein deficiency, on the growth and development of offspring.

Today, we are fortunate that undernutrition isn't a problem for most pregnant women in the United States. However, we now have the opposite problem: approximately 60 percent of women of childbearing age (20 to 39 years old) are overweight or obese. Thus the emphasis of research in the field of nutrition and pregnancy has begun to shift from studying the effects of undernutrition to those of overfeeding. For example, recent research—some of which has come from my laboratory—has revealed that consumption of too much of certain ingredients, like sugars and fats, during pregnancy and nursing may have lasting effects on the baby's body weight, food intake patterns, and other behaviors (more on this in later chapters).

Weight gain is certainly one food-related issue in pregnancy, but there are others. For example, there are often food scares reported in the media, alerting expectant mothers about potential links between a particular food and their baby's well-being. Almost every week there seems to be breaking news about some food additive or ingredient linked to autism, birth defects, and other conditions. Women wonder, *Is this real, or just media hype? Will I get listeriosis from that turkey sandwich I had at the deli before I knew I was pregnant? Was there BPA in that can of soup I had yesterday? Will my child be born with an addiction to caffeine because I had a half-caf latte today? What is DHA, and do I need to take a pill to make sure the baby gets enough of it?* These are just a handful of the anxiety-provoking questions that pregnant women have about food, and a major motivation behind the writing of this book. With mounting evidence regarding the value of good prenatal nutrition, it is important that women who are expecting have the opportunity to learn about the new scientific findings in this area in a realistic, accessible, and hype-free way.

Also, pregnancy can and should be a fun time in life! So instead of being afraid or worrying about the potential bad things that might happen, we can use this information in a positive way. As science tells us more and more about fetal development, we can apply what has been learned to support our growing baby's needs at each step of development. You might have read, or plan to read, other books that describe what development is happening during each week of pregnancy, from those little limbs growing to those fingers and toes taking shape. We know that food is the best medicine and that many of the essential nutrients needed at the various stages of development can be obtained by eating a healthy diet. So in addition to discussing these remarkable milestones,

I will describe the vitamins, minerals, and nutrients that can help support these changes. More on that in Part II.

Being Pregnant Today

Expectant mothers get conflicting messages about eating and weight gain during pregnancy. On the one hand, they are told to forget all the rules and indulge in bonbons while lying on the couch for nine months. On the other hand, they are told to scrutinize their food before consuming it to ensure it won't have any harmful effects on the baby, to avoid gaining too much weight (with no advice on exactly *how* to do that), and then to lose all the baby weight immediately after giving birth (if the celebrities can do it, why can't we?). Between social pressures, hormonal changes, and messages from the media, pregnancy can be hard on a woman's body and body image. Let's try to sort this out.

Eating for Two

Pregnancy is often viewed as a time when women can give in to their food cravings and not worry about their weight. "Eat for two!" and "It's for the baby!" are phrases that mothers-to-be often hear during pregnancy. This type of encouragement can lead women to think that they can pamper themselves by eating anything they want because their body, their baby, or others are telling them to. The belief that it is fine to eat all you want during pregnancy has, unsurprisingly, led to women's eating more. The majority of women in the United States consume more calories per day during their pregnancy than necessary, which may contribute to additional weight gain. Indeed, a recent study at Penn State College of Medicine assessed the differences between overweight and obese women who gained the recommended amount of weight during pregnancy and those who gained too much. The researchers found that women who made less healthy food choices, exercised less, ate more in response to cravings, and described their pregnancy as "eating for two" ended up gaining excessive weight compared to those who were conscious about their eating and exercise habits and did not consume more calories than they needed.

We also tend to pamper expectant mothers during pregnancy because they are in a special state when extra care, attention, and "spoiling" are perceived as beneficial for both the mother and her baby. Throughout pregnancy, many lucky moms-to-be are offered prenatal massages, plenty of rest, and other enjoyable activities. Many also receive extra help around the house from their partners, friends, and relatives, especially during the second half of their pregnancy when certain chores may become especially challenging. All of this is great, and as a society we *should* take care of the people who are producing the next generation of humans! However, when expectant mothers are encouraged to eat more and move less, this self- or society-generated pampering comes at a cost—to both mother and baby.

FOOD FOR THOUGHT

The Institute of Medicine recommends that pregnant women eat *no* extra calories during the first trimester, add 340 extra calories a day in the second trimester, and increase that 340 to about 450 calories a day in the third trimester for a healthy, single baby pregnancy. Even though no extra calories are needed during the first trimester, you may still gain a pound or two during this time (even without consuming more food than usual) because your body is starting to store a little bit of what you eat for the future, when your baby is larger and needs more nutrients. Conversely, you may not gain any weight during the first three months.

Pickles and Ice Cream

Along with the joys of pregnancy can come morning sickness and food cravings. Morning sickness (the common term used to describe the nausea and food aversions that many expectant women experience) can occur throughout a pregnancy, but it is most common in the first trimester. This nausea can alternate with seemingly random and uncontrollable cravings. And there may be some legitimacy behind the stereotype of an expectant mother eating pickles with ice cream at 3 a.m. (after having sent her husband out to the store on an urgent mission to buy it). These cravings can be driven by physiological factors. Cravings are a way of compensating for possible dietary inadequacies and aversions, whereas nausea and vomiting are bodily reactions to abrupt changes in hormone levels. Cravings can also be the result of learning which foods produce feelings of well-being. According to this theory, people have cravings for particular foods because they have learned that when they consume those foods, they feel good. A number of studies also propose that women's diets during pregnancy are strongly influenced by their tastes and eating habits before pregnancy. Thus eating habits, aversions, and cravings that are present before getting pregnant may continue into the pregnancy, possibly in a more pronounced and unrestrained fashion (thanks, hormones!).

Regardless of the causes, both nausea and cravings are a part of pregnancy for many women, and they can have a dramatic effect on appetite. They can limit food choices (particularly if you develop an aversion to entire classes of foods, like meats), which may limit your ability to get essential nutrients that you need for your developing baby. Further, cravings can cause you to go overboard on foods that may not be very healthy for you or the baby (that is, junk food), and this can also lead to more weight gain than intended.

The Skinny on Weight Gain

If the nine-plus months of pregnancy are viewed as a time when social pressures to be slim are somewhat relaxed, then concern about weight gain may be reduced despite an increase in body size. This mentality, combined with socially accepted and expected cravings, may contribute toward gaining more weight than is needed or healthy. U.S. statistics from 2007 show that of those women with an underweight body mass index (BMI), approximately 27 percent gain more weight during their pregnancy than recommended; for women of a normal weight, the figure is 46 percent; for women who were overweight, 59 percent; and for women who were obese, 46 percent. Why might this matter? Studies have found that a higher-than-recommended weight gain is associated with increased weight retention post-pregnancy as well as increased risk for a number of medical conditions that can affect both the mother and the child; these subjects will be covered in greater depth in the upcoming chapters.

To add another layer to this discussion: we live in an increasingly weight-conscious society, which can bring about great confusion and stress for mothers-to-be. Just glancing at the celebrity magazines and tabloids while waiting in line at the supermarket checkout can reveal harsh societal expectations about weight gain during pregnancy. Jessica Simpson and Kim Kardashian, for example, were followed by the press everywhere they went and criticized viciously for gaining "too much" weight while expecting. And then there are the celebrities who seem to lose any and all baby weight immediately after delivery. Brazilian supermodel Gisele Bündchen, for instance, made a big splash in the media when she was photographed on the beach in a bikini just weeks after giving birth, looking very much like she does in the *Sports Illustrated* swimwear issue.

How to Use This Book

As you can see, there are a lot of factors contributing to the confusion about how and what to eat during pregnancy. But ultimately, what is most important is how you can support your baby's development and your own good health during and after pregnancy. I have broken down the information you need to know into three easy parts. Part I covers the basics of *why* it is important to eat well during pregnancy. Chapter 2 reviews the science behind why eating too much (and thereby gaining excess weight) during pregnancy can be a risk factor for complications later on, for you and for your growing baby. Although this book is not exclusively about weight control, it is an issue that affects the majority of women out there, so it warrants being covered in depth. Next, chapter 3 explains which nutrients are most important throughout each of the three trimesters of pregnancy. That way, you can become familiar with these terms, as some of them are on the technical side. So it's okay if you have never heard of choline—I'll explain it and, more important, I'll tell you why you need it and which foods you can get it from naturally.

The fun begins in Part II. Chapters 4, 5, and 6 not only provide you with a week-by-week guide to *what* is happening with your growing baby, but also focus on your needs nutritionally to support the best outcomes for your little one. Each chapter covers a trimester, and each week features a "food of the week" that is high in certain nutrients that are important to consume at that time. There are also recipes and meal prep or snack ideas to go along with each week. Following this week-by-week plan is a great way to not only optimize your nutrition but also test a variety of foods and get creative by trying some fun (yet simple) recipes.

Part III ties everything together and helps you understand *how* you can do this. Let's face it, eating healthy can be a challenge, even when you aren't dealing with raging hormones. Chapters 7 and 8 offer strategies and tips on how you can cope with those pesky hormones, crazy cravings, and other pregnancy-related issues that can make it challenging to eat well. Chapter 9 provides some suggestions for things you can do to get your weight back in check after the baby arrives, and to maintain a healthy eating pattern from here on out—even after the baby is born. Since some of the tips are helpful early on in pregnancy, you may want to jump to Part III while you are working your way week by week through Part II.

At the end of the book you'll find Appendix A, which covers some foods you should avoid as well as the science-based reasons why you should avoid them. It also contains useful information that may help answer questions like whether it is okay to have any alcohol while pregnant (remember that glass you had before you knew?) or why people say you aren't supposed to eat blue cheese. Appendix B reviews what you need to know about eating well while nursing, including foods you may still want to avoid and whether or not you can have a glass or two of wine. Appendix C covers special considerations (like if you are having twins or triplets!) and information about certain health complications that can accompany pregnancy.

* * *

This chapter has covered some of the unique challenges women face today when they become pregnant, and how these challenges can make it difficult to have optimal nutrition during this important developmental period. In chapter 2, we will see in more detail why maintaining a healthy weight during pregnancy is important for not only your own health but also the health of your growing baby.

CHAPTER 2

Why Your Baby Weight Matters

Okay, I'm going to come right out and say it: this is the scary chapter. If you happen to be underweight, overweight, or obese and you are now or are about to become pregnant, some of the information in this chapter may alarm you. I'm not trying to frighten you into gaining or losing weight; rather, I want to share some important research about the relationship between body weight and pregnancy, while underscoring why it is so important to consider what to eat when you are pregnant. While it's true that expectant mothers may have an elevated risk for certain conditions when they are underweight, overweight, or obese, I'm not implying that these conditions *will definitely* occur, but if you happen to fall into one of these weight categories, you are at a higher risk. Fortunately, by changing the way you eat now—with help from the chapters in Part II and the practical tips in Part III—you may be able to lower this risk.

If you are normal weight and don't anticipate that you'll have trouble gaining an amount within the recommended range (see the chart on page 19), you can skip this chapter and get right to the week-by-week recommendations. However, there's been a lot of recent research on the relationship between pre-pregnancy weight and weight gain during pregnancy that I personally find fascinating. So if you're kind of a science and statistics geek like me, keep reading.

Why Do You Have to Worry about Your Weight?

We all know the grim statistics. The rates of overweight and obesity have been increasing in the United States for the past three decades, and it is estimated that by 2030 half the population will be obese. And women of reproductive age are no exception: more than half of all pregnant women in the United States are overweight or obese, and one out of every five women is obese at the start of pregnancy. The situation in other developed countries is equally daunting, with rates similar to those in the United States.

Why the big fuss about weight? Well, we know that being overweight or obese can lead to a plethora of health issues, including increased risk of heart disease, cancer, metabolic syndrome, and depression. However, your prepregnancy weight and the amount of weight you gain during pregnancy can have profound effects on your own *and* your baby's health. Although both issues are important, a woman's prepregnancy weight is sometimes overlooked. However, an increasing number of studies show correlations between a mother's higher weight at conception and negative health effects for her *and* her baby. The following chart outlines some of the conditions that women who are overweight or obese *before* they get pregnant have a higher risk of developing.

There are many reasons why we become overweight or obese. Working women in the Western world have a pretty full plate (no pun intended). Long work hours, financial stress, and unrealistic pressure to keep a perfect home and happy partner can all lead to less time and energy for focusing on our own health and fitness. Hectic schedules can result in an irregular workout regimen (or even a complete lack of exercise) and less-than-optimal nutrition. We cook fewer meals at home because many options for fast and ready-to-eat food are available. And not only do we consume fast food at high rates, but we also eat it quickly. Having less time in general leads to rushed eating, which can contribute to weight gain when the body's fullness response doesn't kick in soon enough to curtail eating. Constant stress can lead to stress eating and overeating, which can also add on extra pounds. These are only some of the factors that contribute to overeating and excess weight gain. With all of this in mind, it is not surprising that, unfortunately, a considerable number of women of childbearing age are entering pregnancy with excess weight.

A DANGEROUS KNOWLEDGE GAP

A recent survey showed that 64 percent of obese women and 40 percent of overweight women overestimated how much weight they should gain during pregnancy. And while many women reported knowing that increased weight can mean an increased risk for pregnancy complications, many were unaware of the specific complications.

The Risks of Being Overweight or Obese before Pregnancy

Condition	Risk	Why It Matters
Preeclampsia: High blood pressure (BP) that develops during pregnancy	2- to 3-fold higher risk	Serious complication that can reduce oxygen and nutrient flow to the baby; your risk is increased for high BP and heart disease years after pregnancy
Gestational diabetes: A form of diabetes that develops during pregnancy	2- to 8-fold higher risk	Risk of developing type 2 diabetes many years later is increased
C-section: Cesarean delivery	2- to 4-fold higher risk	Longer recovery after delivery and increased risk for infections; may not be able to deliver vaginally in future pregnancies
Miscarriage/spontaneous abortion: Loss of fetus before 20th week	1.7-fold greater risk	Loss of a baby; serious emotional trauma
Induction of labor: Administration of hormones to initiate or speed up the labor process if it doesn't start in time (usually by 40 weeks) or does not progress normally	1.7-fold greater risk	May cause more pain; increased risk of needing to have a C-section
Postpartum hemorrhage: Loss of 500 milliliters or more blood after delivery	2-fold greater risk	May need a blood transfusion; leading cause of maternal death
Genital, urinary tract, and wound infections: Infections in these areas post-delivery (either vaginal or C-section delivery)	2-fold greater risk	May increase recovery time and length of hospital stay
Anxiety and depression during pregnancy: Feelings of anxiety, uneasiness, and depressed mood during pregnancy	Greater risk of having increasing levels of anxiety from first to third trimester and higher levels of depression throughout pregnancy	Because of the altered emotional state during pregnancy, risk for postpartum depression may also be increased
Postpartum depression: Prolonged period of emotional disturbance following the birth	2-fold greater risk	Bonding issues and ability to care for the child may be compromised

How Overeating Affects the Baby

Eating too many calories per day or having a diet that's too high in sugar or fat will most likely affect your body both during and after pregnancy. These eating habits will cause you to gain more weight than is needed during pregnancy and make it harder to lose the weight afterward, as well as increase your risk of pregnancy complications. However, maternal overeating may take its largest toll on the baby, who has to cope with a less-than-optimal environment in the womb.

Numerous animal studies have shown that maternal diet can have a long-lasting impact on the offspring's risk of developing mental health disorders, impaired social behaviors, lower cognitive abilities, increased response to stress, and altered reward-related behaviors. For example, a study from my laboratory showed that rat mothers who eat a high-fat diet during pregnancy are likely to have offspring that crave highly palatable food (that is, processed foods engineered to target the brain's most basic pleasure response), which can, in turn, create an intergenerational cycle of eating these types of foods and perhaps perpetuate obesity from one generation to the next. Research in humans suggests that exposure to excess calories, or to gestational diabetes that may have developed as a result of excess food intake, can make a baby grow too large, placing it at risk of having a high birth weight (also known as macrosomia, or "large for gestational age"). Maternal overeating can also influence a child over the long term by increasing the risk of chronic diseases such as obesity and cardiovascular disease, as well as metabolic and psychological disorders in childhood, adolescence, and adulthood. Some studies have even drawn links between prenatal diet and children's intelligence.

How Conditions in the Womb Affect Your Baby

The conditions babies experience in the womb can also have long-lasting effects on their health. The environment that you are exposed to as an expectant mother sends signals to your baby, essentially telling it a story about what life will be like once it is out of the womb. It is hypothesized that this storytelling prepares babies to do well in the world that's being described. This preparation occurs via intricate mechanisms that switch certain of the baby's genes on or off, depending on the story the baby is being told.

If, however, there is a mismatch between the story and the real life the baby encounters outside of the womb, there may be a problem—and quite possibly a big one. For example, if the mother does not eat an adequate diet and/or gain enough weight, the baby may prepare for a life of scarce resources and be born at a low birth weight. The odds that the baby will actually be born into a severe famine are slim in many industrialized societies today, so when a baby is born into a culture characterized by an abundance of food—the exact opposite of what it was "programmed" for—it suddenly has an increased risk for diseases such as diabetes, coronary heart disease, metabolic syndrome, or high blood pressure later in life. That's a high price to pay for a simple mismatch between expectations and reality.

Currently, however, many babies are at an increased risk of being born with a *higher* than normal birth weight (that is, more than 8 pounds 13 ounces, or 4,000 g) and developing into "large for gestational age" infants. In these cases, the growing baby hears the opposite story. Mothers who are overweight or obese prior to getting pregnant or who gain too much weight during pregnancy are preparing their baby for a life that is overabundant with food. But the outcome is often the same: increased obesity and chronic disease risk. While food abundance is generally the case in the Western world, where food availability is often not a concern (although the quality of food available to different socioeconomic groups may vary), the baby who was set up for a food-abundant environment may not thrive, as the prepping for overly plentiful food sources often comes at the price of a disordered metabolic system, a higher proportion of fat tissue at birth, and a higher likelihood that the baby will become obese early on or later in life. Research shows that women who enter their pregnancy overweight or obese, gain excessive weight during pregnancy, or have gestational diabetes, for example, have a greater risk of having a large baby. And further studies show that infants born at a higher than normal body weight have more fat mass and less lean mass compared to average-sized babies, which puts the larger infants at risk for obesity, diabetes, and cardiovascular disease later in life.

WHAT IS A NORMAL BIRTH WEIGHT?

Anywhere between 5.5 and 8.75 pounds is considered a normal birth weight. Less than 5.5 pounds is considered low birth weight; more than 8.8 pounds is considered high birth weight.

How Your Weight Affects Your Baby

There has also been some recent research focused on childhood and adult obesity and how it is affected by the mother's prepregnancy weight and weight gain during pregnancy. Because the rates for both childhood and adult obesity are alarmingly high, scientists are working hard to figure out whether a baby's experience in the womb may be contributing to this epidemic, and if so, how. And so far they've discovered a lot. First, both a mother's prepregnancy body mass index (BMI; see "What Is Body Mass Index [BMI]?", below) and pregnancy weight gain can have a direct effect on a child's BMI in childhood and during the teenage years and can predict adult obesity (the higher one's weight is at any of these ages, the greater the odds that one will be obese as an adult). Second, it is mainly the amount of weight the mother gains during pregnancy that increases this risk of obesity for the child.

In a large study that tracked mothers' prepregnancy BMIs, gestational weight gain, babies' birth weights, and weight throughout childhood and adulthood (up to age 42), researchers found that the more weight mothers gained during pregnancy, the higher the odds were that their children would be obese by the time they were adults. This may be explained by permanent alterations in appetite control as well as hormonal regulation of fat tissue development and metabolism—all of which are programmed while the baby is in the womb and exposed to an excess of nutrients.

WHAT IS BODY MASS INDEX (BMI)? ─────────────────────

BMI is a quick-and-dirty way to figure out where an individual falls on the body weight spectrum. To calculate your own, take your body weight in kilograms (1 pound = 0.45 kilogram) and divide it by your height in meters (1 inch = 0.0254 meter) squared. So if you weigh 130 pounds (58.5 kilograms) and are 5 foot 4 inches (1.625 meters) tall, you divide your weight (58.5) by your height squared (1.625 x 1.625) and get a normal BMI of 22.15. BMI categories are as follows: less than 18.5 = underweight, 18.5 to 24.9 = normal weight, 25 to 29.9 = overweight, and more than 30 = obese. Luckily, you don't have to be a math whiz to figure out your BMI. There are several online tools that you can use to do all of this math for you! Mayoclinic.com and NIH.com have some very user-friendly ones where you just have to enter your height and weight. Note: BMI is just an approximation, and this approach isn't perfect. For example, it does not account for muscle mass. So athletes and people who work out a lot might have a BMI that suggests they are overweight, when in fact they are not.

what to eat when you're pregnant

Maternal obesity, gestational diabetes, and birth weight can also have other health implications. Research shows that large for gestational age babies born to obese mothers and mothers who developed gestational diabetes are at an increased risk for developing metabolic syndrome later in life. Metabolic syndrome is essentially a cluster of increased risk factors for conditions like diabetes, heart disease, and stroke. Another risk of maternal overweight and obesity, as well as excess weight gain during pregnancy, is an increased chance of having to deliver by Cesarean section (or C-section). While there are many maternal risks associated with C-sections, there are also a few—and more long-term—risks for the baby. For example, studies show that babies born via C-section are 33 percent more likely to be overweight or obese later in life compared to babies born vaginally.

WHY THAT TRIP DOWN THE BIRTH CANAL MATTERS ————

Some people have postulated a hygiene hypothesis: that the increased risk for being overweight or obese later in life among infants born via C-section may stem from their missing out on an essential element bestowed during vaginal birth. On a baby's way through the birth canal, it is normally exposed to maternal and intestinal bacteria. Babies delivered via Cesarean section miss this exposure; they are exposed directly to nonmaternal bacteria from the external environment. This early-life difference in germ exposure and acquisition could have long-lasting effects on the baby's gut microbe environment and various disorders related to it (of which there are many, including overweight and obesity later in life). We're only now starting to understand the importance of all those helpful bugs in our gut.

In addition to physical health outcomes, a number of mental health–related outcomes have been associated with maternal weight status and gestational weight gain, such as ADHD, autism, anxiety, depression, learning disabilities, impulsivity, and even Parkinson's and Alzheimer's diseases later in life. For instance, mothers who were obese prior to becoming pregnant were found to be twice as likely to have children with issues relating to emotional intensity, as well as problems regulating sadness, fear, and anger. Recent scientific evidence also suggests a link between maternal obesity and childhood ADHD, with some studies showing that obese mothers are twice as likely to have children with ADHD compared to mothers with a normal BMI, and that the risk for childhood ADHD is increased if the mother is obese prior to becoming pregnant. Scientists hypothesize that one way these two issues may be related is through hormonal dysfunctions that occur as the fetus is developing inside the womb. Maternal diabetes has also been linked to psychological problems in children, with children of diabetic mothers having higher rates of ADHD symptoms and hyperactivity and increased risk for anxiety, depression, and trouble with social situations.

THE LINK BETWEEN PREGNANCY
WEIGHT GAIN AND AUTISM

Obesity, hypertension, and consuming too much of a high-fat diet during pregnancy may increase a child's risk of mental health disorders such as autism. Rates of autism in the United States have been rising right alongside obesity rates. One mechanism by which obesity may be linked to the development of autism is through a hormone called leptin. Leptin is released in proportion to one's body fat, so in cases of maternal obesity, babies are exposed to higher amounts of the hormone while in the womb. These higher exposures can lead to dysfunctions of the placenta and disruption of normal brain development, perhaps leading to autism or autism spectrum disorders. In addition, inadequate maternal intake of folic acid and certain healthful dietary fats has been associated with autism in children, with studies showing reduced incidence of autism with folic acid supplementation and increased rates in children whose mothers consumed little omega-3 fatty acids.

One final point to consider is that the health effects associated with maternal obesity and excessive weight gain during pregnancy not only may be lifelong but also may be intergenerational, meaning they may potentially affect your grandchildren and great-grandchildren. It makes sense: babies exposed to excessive calories in the womb can become obese adults, once again predisposing the next generation to a greater chance of obesity.

How Much Weight *Should* You Gain During Pregnancy?

At this point, you may be thinking, *Well, I have to gain* some *weight, so how much should I gain to have a healthy pregnancy and baby?* You may have already heard many different answers to this question. When more than 1,000 women were surveyed as part of a study in 1999, researchers found that many were actually advised by health care professionals to gain more or less weight during pregnancy than the Institute of Medicine recommends. And nearly one-third weren't given any advice about weight gain at all. Aside from demonstrating that discrepancies exist between advice offered by health care professionals and the official guidelines, this study also illustrates the importance of having accurate information, since advised and "target" weight gains (how much weight women believed they *should* gain while pregnant) were associated with how much weight the women *actually* gained. A more recent study of medical records conducted in 2010 found that doctors and expectant women discussed prepregnancy body weight only 11 percent of the time, and discussions about weight gain during pregnancy were indicated only 15 percent of the time, demonstrating a need for accurate information and awareness around this topic—especially considering the health risks associated with high prepregnancy weight and too much or too little weight gain during pregnancy.

When discussing ideal pregnancy weight gain, remember that although there are general guidelines, there is no one magic number that fits everyone. The weight gain that is best for you is based on your prepregnancy BMI (see chart), which is why the number of pounds that your mom or your friend gained during her pregnancy may not be the right amount for you (so don't even ask).

Recommended Single Pregnancy Weight Gain for Each BMI Category

If you start your pregnancy as . . .	You should gain . . .
Underweight: BMI less than 18.5	28 to 40 pounds
Normal Weight: BMI 18.5 to 24.9	25 to 35 pounds
Overweight: BMI 25.0 to 29.9	15 to 25 pounds
Obese (includes all classes): BMI greater than or equal to 30.0	11 to 20 pounds

Source: Institute of Medicine.

IT'S TWINS: CAN I DOUBLE THE WEIGHT?

According to the Institute of Medicine, if you're pregnant with twins, you need to gain significantly more weight compared to a one-baby pregnancy:

If you start your pregnancy as...	You should gain...
Normal weight: BMI of 18.5 to 24.9	37 to 54 pounds
Overweight: BMI of 25 to 29.9	31 to 51 pounds
Obese: BMI over 30	24 to 42 pounds

Note: Neither the Institute of Medicine nor the American Pregnancy Association offer guidelines on how much weight to gain with twins if you are underweight. If this is your situation, it is best to discuss it with your doctor, but plan on gaining at least 40 pounds.

Weight gain during pregnancy provides nourishment for the developing baby and allows your body to store additional nutrients for breastfeeding after delivery. Putting this weight on slowly and steadily is best, because your baby requires a daily supply of nutrients that come from the foods you eat. However, you should not worry or give yourself a hard time if you gain a little less or a little more than is recommended in a given week. You may gain a bit more during some weeks and less in others, which can result in the same total weight gain at the end. However, if you find yourself suddenly gaining or losing more weight than you should (especially in the third trimester), you should contact your health care provider, as it may be a sign of complications.

WHERE DOES THE WEIGHT GO?

As your weight increases, you may be wondering where all those pounds are accumulating. As it turns out, they're added to many places throughout the body, with, of course, some variation among women, the chart on the next page shows the approximate amounts and locations.

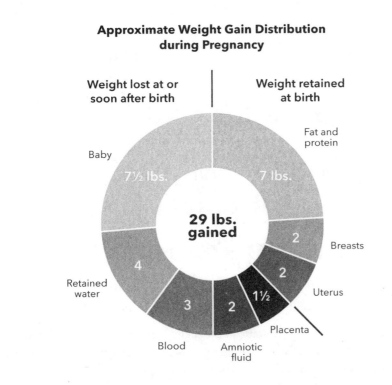

**Approximate Weight Gain Distribution
during Pregnancy**

Weight lost at or
soon after birth

Weight retained
at birth

Baby

Fat and
protein

7½ lbs.

7 lbs.

29 lbs.
gained

2

Breasts

4

2

Retained
water

1½

Uterus

3

2

Placenta

Blood

Amniotic
fluid

Source: Adapted from www.marchofdimes.org/pregnancy/weight-gain-during-pregnancy.aspx.

* * *

Okay, enough with the doom and gloom. I warned you at the beginning of this chapter that many of these statistics and studies might seem scary. I wanted to include this information so you would understand how important it is to maintain a healthy weight during pregnancy. Now that you know how much weight you are supposed to gain and why too much (or even too little) can be potentially harmful for you and your baby, it's time to change gears. In the chapters that follow, I use science to our advantage and talk about what you *can do*—week by week—to help program your belly for the best. Just as being overweight or eating an unhealthy diet can put you and your growing baby at risk, you can also capitalize on what we know about the benefits of certain nutrients during fetal development to help your baby thrive while keeping your own weight in check. So now let's talk about all the incredible (and tasty and satisfying) foods you *can* eat to support your baby's healthy development and growth.

CHAPTER 3

The Key Nutrients You Need during Pregnancy

Throughout the nine-plus months of pregnancy, the baby relies entirely on its mother's daily nutrient intake and body stores for healthy growth and development. Baby's little fingers, toes, eyes, and nose, as well as its nervous system and all other organ systems, are forming and require a continuous supply of building blocks for the ongoing construction. For you, its mother, consuming nutritious foods and gaining a healthy amount of weight during pregnancy are essential to support this growth.

In this chapter, I outline the specific types of vitamins, minerals, and nutrients that are most crucial for supporting the changes of pregnancy. I'm going to spend some time describing what each of these nutrients is and does, because although you have probably heard about some of them, unless you were a nutrition major you probably don't remember what they actually do. (For the sake of simplicity, the term "nutrient" is used throughout the book to describe macronutrients, such as fats, protein, and carbohydrates, as well as vitamins and minerals.)

Also, I will review why you and your baby need these nutrients, and the best places to get them. In the chapters that follow this one, I'll give you a detailed plan to incorporate foods that are rich in these nutrients into your diet and tell you week by week when they are especially important to consume. Let's get started!

Now that you're pregnant and need to support a rapidly growing embryo within a not-yet-visible belly, you may be wondering whether it's time to start eating for two. The answer is no. This may be surprising and contrary to what your mother, your friends, and others have told you, but as I mentioned in the last chapter, you actually don't need to eat *any* extra calories during the first trimester. It is important, however, to be sure that you are getting the appropriate amount of calories based on your BMI (see box on page 16), age, and activity level. For example, if you are between 31 and 50 years old and have a BMI of 21.5 (within the normal range), you need 1,800 to 2,400 calories per day depending on your level of physical activity. To find out how many calories you specifically need each day, enter your age, weight, height, gender, and physical activity information into an online calculator or a calorie calculator app, such as Lose It! by Fit Now, Calorie Counter & Diet Tracker by MyFitnessPal, or Calorie Counter PRO by MyNetDiary.

The Key Nutrients

Based on the knowledge that certain bodily systems develop during specific weeks of pregnancy, we can optimize our nutrition by consuming, during particular time periods, foods that are rich in the nutrients that support this growth. The key nutrients described here are important during *all three trimesters* of pregnancy, but I have also noted whether some are more important during specific trimesters. You'll notice that several more nutrients are discussed for the first trimester than for the second and third trimesters. That is because so much of your baby's most intricate and specific development occurs during this early phase. During the first trimester, cells undergo rapid differentiation, becoming more specialized and able to carry out the specific functions of the organs they belong to. Further, developmental risks are highest in the first three months, so optimal nutrition during this period is essential. However, don't feel you should abandon the nutrients emphasized here once the first trimester is complete—they are helpful for supporting proper growth throughout your pregnancy.

Folate/Folic Acid (also known as Vitamin B9)

What you need: 600 mcg of dietary folate equivalents (DFEs—see sidebar on page 24) per day (500 mcg per day during breastfeeding)

Why you need it: You may already be familiar with this nutrient, as it is recommended for all women of childbearing age regardless of pregnancy status. Folic acid (which is what we call the synthetic form present in supplements or fortified foods) or folate (the natural form present in foods) is a B vitamin (B9) involved in making and repairing DNA as well as aiding in numerous biological reactions. It is absolutely crucial in cell division, which is why adequate intake is so important early on in pregnancy, when the most rapid growth is occurring, with all of those little cells dividing and multiplying.

Adequate folate sources are also needed to prevent neural tube defects (such as spina bifida and anencephaly)—the most serious complication of folic acid deficiency, which can cause abnormalities in the baby's brain and spinal cord. The neural tube forms and closes very early on in pregnancy (closure is complete at about 4 weeks), so daily intake of folate or folic acid before conception and during the first month of pregnancy is critical. And there is some evidence that taking a folic acid supplement before conception and early on in pregnancy can reduce the risk of autism in children, further underscoring the importance of this vitamin during the very early stages of pregnancy. Last, recent research has also shown that obese women metabolize folate differently from normal weight women. In the previous chapter it was mentioned that increased weight has been associated with increased risk for neural tube defects; that may be because less folate may be available to babies of obese women.

You may have also heard about concerns regarding a link between folic acid and cancer. Here's what you need to know: recent animal research has found that folic acid supplementation increases the risk of breast cancer tumors in offspring exposed to a carcinogen. Folate is known to be necessary for the division of cells, and cancerous cells are no exception; thus it has been said that, with respect to cancer, folate may protect against initiation of cancer, but promote proliferation. That said, unless you *have* cancer, it is wise to take folate, given all of its health benefits.

WHAT IS A DFE?

Folate intake is expressed in dietary folate equivalents, or DFEs, because food-based folate and folic acid from supplements are not absorbed in the same way. One mcg of food-based folate equals 0.6 mcg of folic acid from supplements or fortified foods (if consumed with food) and 0.5 mcg of folic acid (if consumed on an empty stomach). In the United States, the recommended daily intake is 400 DFEs before pregnancy and 600 DFEs once you are pregnant.

Where you get it: To get your daily dose, you could eat about 2½ cups of steamed spinach or cooked kidney beans. It turns out that we absorb folic acid more efficiently than folate from foods. However, that does not mean you should rely entirely on a folic acid supplement. Regularly consuming foods that are naturally high in folate or supplemented with folic acid can supply you with adequate or near-adequate amounts of the vitamin if you know where to look for it. The best source of folate is dark leafy greens, such as kale, collard greens, dandelion leaves, and spinach. Vegetables and citrus fruits, legumes, nuts and seeds, dairy products, eggs, grains, and seafood are also good options. Because natural folate is sensitive to heat, it is best to eat your veggies and fruit fresh and raw; for example, as part of a smoothie. However, if you do steam or boil your veggies, grains, or legumes, be sure to retain the water, because folate is soluble in water, and that's where it will be. You can use the leftover water to make a soup (freeze it in ice-cube trays if you aren't making one right away). Or, if you are making baby food, use it to thin out baby's pureed veggies.

FOOD THAT IS ALREADY FORTIFIED

The United States started fortifying our food supply with folic acid in 1998 (as did some other countries at varying dates). Folic acid is now present in all enriched white flour (added along with other vitamins, as required by law) and many flour-containing foods such as breads and cereals, which has helped to dramatically reduce the number of babies born with neural tube defects. However, many people are now avoiding gluten, and if you are one of them, it's especially important to make sure you're getting the recommended amount of folate from gluten-free sources.

Should you take a folic acid supplement? The current international recommendation is to take a folic acid supplement from the first moment you begin trying to conceive through 12 weeks of pregnancy. However, recommendations tend to vary from one source to another and even from doctor to doctor. Speak to your health care provider about taking folic acid supplements beyond the first trimester, especially if you're eating plenty of leafy greens or foods fortified with folic acid, as it may not be necessary to supplement. As with most things in life, too much of a good thing can be bad; higher folate levels in expectant mothers (measured at 28 weeks) have been shown to correlate with increased fat and insulin resistance in their children at age 6.

If you're taking a folic acid supplement, or if your prenatal multivitamin contains folic acid, make sure that your intake of vitamins B6 and B12 is adequate. If there isn't a proper balance among these vitamins, fetal growth can be reduced. In fact, a recent study showed that women who took a folic acid supplement in the third trimester were more likely to have lower birth weight infants who also had an increased weight gain in the first month of life. While increased weight gain after birth in lower birth weight infants might seem like a good thing, it actually isn't, because it has been linked to obesity and obesity-related disorders later in life.

Vitamin B12

What you need: 2.6 mcg per day (2.8 mcg per day during breastfeeding)

Why you need it: Vitamin B12 (also known as cobalamin) is closely related to folate and is crucial for brain and nervous system development, blood formation, and numerous other actions that take place in just about every cell of your baby's growing body. As with folic acid, being deficient in B12 can increase the risk of neural tube defects. Research shows that low levels of B12 early in pregnancy increase the risk of neural tube defects nearly threefold, whereas adequate intake of B12 has a 72-percent protective effect against these defects. Also, optimal intake of vitamin B12 (in addition to folate and B6) may reduce the risk of cleft lip and palate in your baby. In fact, taking a daily B12 supplement in addition to folic acid at least 3 months before conception and for the first 3 months of pregnancy—if you are or may be vitamin B12 deficient—may also prevent the risk of neural tube defects better than taking folic acid alone. There is a biochemical explanation for this: without adequate levels of B12, folate can't be metabolized appropriately and used by the cells. Finally, research has shown an association between low maternal vitamin B12 during pregnancy and insulin resistance in children at age 6, highlighting the importance of adequate nutrient intake for both the short- and the long-term health of your baby.

Where you get it: If you are an omnivore, you can easily get all the B12 you need from your diet. Great sources of B12 include meat, fish (such as cod or salmon), dairy products (milk, cheese), and eggs. Just 3 ounces of cooked salmon contains 4.8 mcg (which is more than enough!); so does 3 ounces of broiled beef sirloin (1.4 mcg) and 1 cup of low-fat milk (1.2 mcg).

Vitamin B12 is found only in animal products, which is why supplementing is of particular importance if you are vegan or a vegetarian
who doesn't regularly eat eggs or dairy, as you may be lacking the
vitamin in your diet, in which case you should consult your physician
and may need to take vitamin B12 supplements or shots.

Zinc

What you need: 11 mg per day (12 mg per day during breastfeeding)

Why you need it: Zinc is an essential mineral that your baby needs for its
rapidly dividing cells and protein and DNA synthesis, as well as many other
developments. There is some evidence that adequate zinc intake can be beneficial for you as well (and by extension, even more beneficial for your baby).
Recent research shows that optimal zinc intake in first-time mothers may
reduce the risk of developing gestational hypertension (onset of high blood
pressure in pregnancy). While severe zinc deficiencies are rare in the United
States, according to the World Health Organization, more than 80 percent
of pregnant women worldwide have inadequate zinc intake. This statistic
suggests that even if you don't have symptoms of zinc deficiency (such as
suppressed appetite, growth retardation, and reduced immune function, which
often are present only in severe deficiency), you may still be consuming less
zinc than recommended.

Where you get it: Just 3 ounces of cooked Alaskan king crab (6.5 mg) and
1 cup of canned baked beans with no salt added (5.8 mg) provides all the zinc
you need. Fortunately, you can get all the zinc you need fairly easily from your
diet. Good sources of zinc include fortified breakfast cereals, lamb, ground
beef, turkey, Alaskan king crab, tofu, pumpkin seeds, garbanzo and kidney
beans, wheat germ, whole grains, yogurt, milk, almonds, and collard greens,
just to name a few! Zinc supplements are not recommended, due to limited
data that they provide any benefit.

We absorb less zinc from nonanimal sources, which may be a
concern if you're vegan or vegetarian. However, you can increase
the amount of zinc you absorb by soaking and cooking legumes
and combining plant-based zinc sources with acidic ingredients
such as lemon juice.

Vitamin B6

What you need: 1.9 mg per day (2 mg per day during breastfeeding)

Why you need it: Vitamin B6, also known as pyridoxine, is another important B vitamin that helps your body metabolize macronutrients such as proteins, carbohydrates, and fat. It also helps to form new red blood cells, is involved in your baby's brain and nervous system development by making neurotransmitters (brain chemicals), and contributes to numerous other actions. Research also shows that adequate vitamin B6 levels before conception and early in pregnancy may help to prevent pregnancy loss. Furthermore, vitamin B6 has been long known to help alleviate nausea and vomiting, which means it will be your friend if you fall victim to morning sickness (more on that in the next chapter).

Where you get it: If you eat 1 cup of canned chickpeas (1.1 mg), 1 cup of boiled potatoes (0.4 mg), and 1 medium banana (0.4 mg), you've gotten your full daily requirement of vitamin B6. Taking a B6 supplement is not necessary, as you can easily get all the vitamin B6 you need through your diet. B6 is widely available in a variety of foods, good sources of which are baked potatoes, salmon, chicken, cooked spinach, prune juice, chickpeas, brown rice, bananas, avocados, and pork loin, among many others. If you're taking a prenatal vitamin, it likely has 100 percent of the daily dose of B6, which, in addition to the many vitamin B6–rich foods you may be consuming as part of your normal diet, provides you with a more than adequate daily dose of the vitamin. A mild excess of B6 is unlikely to cause any negative effects for you or your baby, and supplementation above the daily recommended dose has been used for decades to treat nausea in pregnant women. Research shows that doses of 50 mg or more per day during the first trimester do not produce detrimental effects. However, it is important to note that the Institute of Medicine did establish an upper limit for vitamin B6 of 100mg/day.

A SPECIAL NEED FOR B6

A recent study found that compared to their nonobese counterparts, pregnant women with obesity had significantly lower levels of vitamin B6, perhaps accounting in part for some of the health complications associated with maternal obesity discussed in chapter 2.

Magnesium

What you need: If you are between ages 19 and 30: 350 mg per day (310 mg per day during breastfeeding). If you are between ages 31 and 50: 360 mg per day (320 mg per day during breastfeeding).

what to eat when you're pregnant

Why you need it: Magnesium is beneficial for both you and your baby during pregnancy. In fact, more than 300 enzymes in your baby's body require magnesium for normal functioning. Additionally, because magnesium aids in tissue repair, its deficiency may lead to preeclampsia (high blood pressure beginning in the second or third trimester of pregnancy), which is why it's important to consume adequate amounts of it early on. Magnesium also helps your muscles to relax, and optimum magnesium levels throughout pregnancy may help prevent leg cramps and even premature contractions and preterm birth. And your tired muscles will appreciate any extra relaxation!

Where you get it: One ounce of dry-roasted almonds (80 mg), ½ cup of boiled spinach (78 mg), 1 packet of instant oatmeal (36 mg), ½ cup of cooked black beans (60 mg), ½ cup of cooked brown rice (42 mg), 3 ounces of roasted chicken breast (22 mg), and 1 cup of cubed avocado (44 mg). As you can see, it's not hard to get all the magnesium you need from your diet. Other good sources include pumpkin and sunflower seeds, salmon, halibut, wheat germ, bran cereal, quinoa, cashews, soybeans, tofu, baked potato (with skin), yogurt, and many others.

Choline

What you need: 450 mg per day (550 mg per day during breastfeeding)

Why you need it: Choline is an important nutrient for pregnancy and appears to be particularly important early on. As with folic acid and vitamin B12, adequate choline intake prior to conception and early in pregnancy is associated with a lower risk of neural tube defects. Choline is integral for building cells in your growing baby, as well as for healthy brain development. In fact, choline can have long-term effects on your baby's brain development, cognitive abilities, and memory, and may even reduce its risk of cognitive decline decades down the road. Some animal research suggests that adequate choline intake during pregnancy may possibly even counteract some of the detrimental effects of alcohol consumption. While it is unclear whether this applies to humans, nor is it a green light to drink choline cosmos, this finding does provide further evidence that choline can be beneficial during pregnancy. In addition to being beneficial for your baby, choline can have positive effects for you. Studies show that adequate choline intake can reduce your risk of breast cancer and potentially lower the risk of some other chronic diseases such as heart disease. And as it does for your baby, choline may boost your brainpower!

Where you get it: Two large hard-boiled eggs (226 mg), ½ cup of firm tofu (35 mg), 4 ounces of cooked cod (80 mg), 1 tablespoon of brewer's yeast

(60 mg), and ½ cup of cooked kidney beans (54 mg). Choline is abundant in a variety of foods, and unless you think you're falling short, you likely don't need a supplement. Wheat germ, broccoli, quinoa, milk, spinach, potatoes, chicken, navy beans and soybeans, fish, and nuts are some additional great sources.

WHAT ABOUT ORGANIC?

We hear a lot about the dangers of pesticides, hormones, and genetically modified organisms (GMOs) in our food. Do you need to worry *more* about this now that you are pregnant? Maybe. A study published in July 2014 examined the health benefits associated with the consumption of organic foods during pregnancy, and found that women who ate organic produce "often" or "mostly" had a significantly lower risk of preeclampsia during pregnancy.

By United States Department of Agriculture (USDA) standards, organic crops are free from pesticides, GMOs, synthetic fertilizers, irradiation, and sewage sludge. For organic livestock, antibiotics or growth hormones are not used and animals are fed organic feed. Pesticides such as persistent organic pollutants (POPs) are of particular interest because they can accumulate in our bodies due to their chemical stability, long half lives, and overall resistance to degradation. We get POPs in our systems through diet, and studies have shown that mothers can pass on POPs to a developing fetus through the placenta or postnatally through breast milk. However, is this second-hand exposure necessarily cause for alarm? It seems that it is.

A recent study that measured pesticide exposure in a group of pregnant women looked at whether or not this has an effect on fetal development and gestational age. The researchers found that women with higher levels of HCB (hexachlorobenzene) and PCBs (polychlorinated biphenyls) had lower birth weight babies than other women. The researchers also noted that the association was seen more often in women with inadequate or excessive weight gain during pregnancy, making it difficult to draw a substantial conclusion. However, another study published in 2014 measured preconception levels of POPs in both the mother and the father and found a significant association between POP concentration and lower birth weight. This is concerning because low birth weight is associated with several medical complications.

Few studies have been done regarding the use of hormone injections and antibiotics in livestock, but one study that was published in 2007 attempted to uncover possible long-term risks associated with their use. When livestock are slaughtered, not all of the steroids (or antibiotics) have necessarily been fully metabolized and remain in the muscles, fat, and other organs. Researchers have shown that a mother who eats a lot of beef while pregnant significantly impacts her son's sperm concentration, which is in line with previous research showing that perinatal exposure to steroid hormones can induce testicular dysgenesis syndrome, resulting in many different testicular problems, such as low sperm count.

So what should you do? If possible, try to buy organic meats, poultry, fruits, and vegetables. Although organic food tends to cost more money, it is well worth the investment.

Iron

What you need: 27 mg per day (9 mg per day during breastfeeding)

Why you need it: Iron is key during pregnancy. It helps your body make hemoglobin, which is needed for your blood to carry oxygen. It is also needed for supplying your muscles with oxygen and maintaining a healthy immune system. While you may have been extensively advised to take an iron supplement starting even before pregnancy or may be taking one now, the research regarding the benefits to the baby and to you of daily iron supplementation during the first trimester is actually quite mixed. An extensive review of studies did not find any health benefits for either the mother or the baby with iron supplementation of 30 to 40 mg/day (the routinely recommended dose for iron-replete women during pregnancy) in women who were *not* iron-deficient.

Where you get it: One serving of breakfast cereal (fortified with 100 percent of your daily value [DV] of iron, which is 18 mg), ½ cup of boiled and drained spinach (3 mg), 1 medium baked potato with skin (2 mg), ½ cup of firm tofu (3 mg), and 18 oil-roasted cashew nuts (2 mg). There are two types of iron—heme and non-heme iron. Heme iron comes only from animal sources, such as meats, fish, seafood (clams contain nearly 14 mg in a 3-ounce serving!), and poultry. It is the better-absorbed form of iron, with an absorption rate of approximately 15 to 35 percent. Non-heme iron can be found in both animal and plant foods; it is found in fortified cereals, eggs, milk, pumpkin seeds, lentils and other legumes, spinach, and prune juice. However, the majority of the iron in these foods is poorly absorbed. Not to worry, though! You can bump up your non-heme iron absorption by eating foods rich in vitamin C alongside the non-heme-iron sources, such as having lentils with red bell peppers, or indulging in a fresh fruit dessert after a legume meal—strawberries, papayas, kiwi, oranges, cantaloupe, and guava are all packed with vitamin C!

FOODS THAT ENHANCE OR INHIBIT IRON ABSORPTION ———

Certain foods can increase your non-heme iron absorption, whereas others will prevent your gut from taking in what little iron there is in a given bean, veggie, or other non-heme iron source.

Absorption enhancers:

- Vitamin C can nearly triple the rate of absorption

- Heme iron sources such as meats, fish, and seafood

Absorption inhibitors:

- Phytic acid that is present in plant foods (such as grains and legumes)

- Fiber

- Coffee and tea (tannic acid in tea)

- Calcium, zinc, magnesium, copper

- Egg protein (in whites and in yolk)

- Some herbs. If you're an avid tea drinker, be sure to moderate your intake of chamomile, peppermint, feverfew, and St. John's wort teas, as they can lower your iron absorption rate. If you're unsure about a certain herb, always consult your doctor.

While iron supplements undoubtedly help you build up your body's iron stores—which will be most important during the second and third trimesters—some studies suggest that iron supplementation may do more harm than good, especially if you're starting out with an adequate iron status before pregnancy. A large-scale review of numerous trials involving more than twenty-seven thousand women showed that while iron supplementation in pregnancy did decrease the risk of anemia, iron deficiency in pregnancy, and giving birth to a low-weight baby, it was also associated with numerous and sometimes nasty side effects, such as constipation and other gastrointestinal issues like nausea, vomiting, diarrhea, and an increased risk of high hemoglobin levels in the mother at term. Research also shows that taking iron supplements during pregnancy if you're not iron-deficient can increase your risk of gestational diabetes and preeclampsia, thus putting both you and your baby at risk for short- and long-term complications. Furthermore, iron supplements are well known to induce nausea—and if you're already experiencing morning sickness, the last thing you want is to take something that might make things worse.

If you're taking an iron supplement but it makes you so nauseous that you can't eat anything else, then consider the risks and benefits associated with the consumption of one nutrient versus a deficiency of many more. Because of these concerns, it may be a good idea to first get your blood iron (serum ferritin) level checked out, and then follow your doctor's advice regarding whether or not iron supplementation is necessary.

IRON SUPPLEMENTATION IN THE THIRD TRIMESTER

Although iron supplementation in the first and second trimesters may not be a good idea, in the third trimester it may be appropriate to introduce a supplement if you're finding it hard to maintain an adequate intake of iron-rich foods, or if you're iron-deficient or anemic. Iron levels decrease significantly from the beginning until toward the end of pregnancy. However, the third trimester is also the time when your baby is pulling iron from your diet and body stores to use for the first six months of life. Your doctor will check for anemia early on in the third trimester (or late in the second trimester). A hemoglobin level below 110 g/L (11 g/dL) or a hematocrit level below 6.83 mmol/L (0.33 L/L; 33 percent) are considered anemic during pregnancy. Although mild anemia is considered normal during pregnancy, if you are anemic or close to anemic, you should discuss with your doctor whether you might benefit from adding an iron supplement to your diet. In addition, remember that taking a supplement on an empty stomach and with a glass of orange juice (or another source of vitamin C) will increase your iron absorption.

Omega-3 Fatty Acids: EPA and DHA

What you need: 500 or more mg per day of omega-3 fatty acids EPA and DHA, of which 300 mg or more are from DHA (same amounts during breastfeeding)

Why you need it: Numerous studies show health benefits from consuming EPA and DHA (the two main omega-3 fatty acids), with higher intakes associated with healthy brain development, improved memory, and improved cognitive and intellectual abilities in childhood and later in life. The clearest benefits are in prevention of premature birth, which affects brain development; babies born at full term have better-developed nervous systems. In addition, recent research shows a link between omega-3 fatty acid consumption and allergy risk in children as they grow up, with decreased allergy risk linked to higher maternal fish consumption.

DHA is one of the omega-3 fatty acids that you may have heard about, particularly with respect to its importance during pregnancy. It is highly beneficial for your baby's brain and vision and is especially key in the third trimester, when rapid brain growth occurs. Higher maternal levels of DHA have been associated with beneficial cognitive development outcomes in children, such as better attention span, visual acuity, and sleep in infants. In addition to its known role in improving brain and vision development, studies show that adequate intake of DHA from foods may lead to a healthier body fat ratio and insulin sensitivity in the infant at birth. Taking DHA supplements has also been shown to modestly increase gestation duration and infant size at birth, which can be helpful when trying to prevent having a preterm or low-birth-weight baby.

EPA is another key omega-3 fatty acid, highly related to DHA. It helps the baby absorb DHA. It is therefore beneficial to have an adequate intake of both fatty acids, and not just DHA. Fortunately, many foods that contain DHA often also have EPA—making your life easier!

WHICH FISH ARE CONSIDERED SAFE TO EAT? ─────────────

While some fish contain high levels of methylmercury and poly-chlorinated biphenyls (which are just as harmful as they are hard to pronounce), there are plenty of fish in the sea that are safe for both you and your baby. These include salmon (wild-caught, not farmed), sardines, herring, trout, Atlantic and Pacific mackerel, anchovies, canned light tuna, shrimp, pollock, and catfish.

DHA supplementation during pregnancy, especially in the second half, has been associated with beneficial effects. If you're not eating enough fish, eggs, and other DHA-rich sources, consider adding a supplement.

Where you get it: Three ounces of salmon can contain between 700 and 1,800 mg of omega-3s (EPA and DHA), 500 to 1,400 mg of which is from DHA. The general recommendation is to consume fatty fish at least twice a week (up to 12 ounces) from safe food sources (that is, fish low in mercury, with less than 0.05 parts per billion of mercury in one serving of fish). Don't fancy fish? No problem. Other sources of EPA and DHA are now available, such as DHA-enriched eggs, purified fish and algal supplements, grass-fed beef, and fortified milk and yogurt. However, it may still be difficult to get the recommended amount of DHA and EPA from fortified foods and the recommended two servings of fish or seafood per week. Two weekly servings of fish provide only about 100 to 250 mg of omega-3 fatty acids per day (although amounts vary—some fish, such as salmon, have much more EPA and DHA than others),

what to eat when you're pregnant

of which 50 to 100 mg is from DHA, and plant-based oils supply minuscule amounts of EPA and no DHA, leading to a total EPA and DHA amount that is much lower than recommended. It may therefore be a good idea to consider adding a supplement to your diet. In addition, if you're vegan or vegetarian, you very likely need to supplement your diet to provide adequate amounts of EPA and DHA for your baby's developing brain, as your diet is naturally lacking in these nutrients. It is still unclear whether enough EPA and DHA can be made by your body if you have an adequate intake of alpha-linoleic acid (ALA)—another major omega-3 fatty acid that is found in plants, such as nuts, oils, and certain greens.

STAY ON THE SAFE SIDE

Even though fatty fish are great sources of DHA and other omega-3 fatty acids, it may be a good idea to alternate between eating fish, fortified eggs, and algae, and consider taking a supplement to make sure that you get all the DHA you need. I say this because it is recommended that pregnant women consume only up to 12 ounces of fish per week due to pollutants found in fish, such as mercury.

That said, animal foods, especially fish and eggs, are great sources of DHA. Salmon, catfish, canned light tuna, anchovies, herring, halibut, fish oil, and fortified eggs are all excellent options for sourcing this nutrient. And luckily there is a lot of overlap between the foods rich in vitamin D and those containing DHA, so you're likely to easily double up when choosing fatty fish or eggs.

BABY'S DEVELOPMENT IN THE SECOND TRIMESTER

Over the course of these three months, your baby grows from two ounces to nearly two pounds. The nutrients that were essential in the first trimester remain key; however, a few extra ones should be added to your list to accommodate the specific growth and development occurring at this time. Your baby's tissues (bone, teeth, hair, skin, nails, blood, fat, and muscle) and organs and organ systems (digestive and immune systems, reproductive organs) are developing and maturing; this makes extra protein, fatty acids, iron, calcium, and other vitamins and minerals crucial during this period. In addition, your baby is acquiring new abilities such as hearing, reacting to light, wiggling, kicking, and even thumb-sucking! With your morning sickness likely gone or fading (more on coping with morning sickness in chapter 4), it may be easier to focus on receiving optimal nutrition now than it was at the beginning of your pregnancy.

Protein

What you need: 1.1 g per kilogram of body weight, or roughly 75 to 100 g of protein per day (same amounts during breastfeeding)

Why you need it: Your protein needs are significantly increased during pregnancy, especially during the second and third trimesters. Proteins are made of amino acids, the building blocks of both your baby's cells and growing body as well as your own expanding tissues that accommodate your baby's growth. In addition, proteins serve as cell-to-cell communicators, are involved in immune system functioning, and act as enzymes, aiding in thousands of chemical reactions. With a lot of action happening now and in the next trimester in terms of your baby's and your own body's growth, your protein needs are higher than when you're not expecting.

ARE ALL PROTEINS THE SAME?

While most people have no problem getting enough protein, it is important to note that not all protein is the same. Consuming *complete* or high-quality protein can be tricky. *Complete protein* sources are foods that contain all the essential amino acids (amino acids are the building blocks of protein, and there are nine essential ones) in "perfect" proportions—in amounts that are most optimal for your body to support its functions. The essential amino acids are called *essential* because you need to get them from your diet, as your body cannot make them (unlike the nonessential amino acids). Most animal foods (for example, eggs, milk, cheese, fish, poultry, and meat) have complete protein, whereas plant foods (such as nuts, seeds, grains, and beans) tend to lack one or more amino acids. Does that mean that you should focus only on animal foods? No. You can get all the protein you need by eating plant foods alone *if* you eat a variety. While they are considered incomplete because they lack one or more of the essential amino acids, combining complementary proteins (two or more protein sources that together contain all the essential amino acids, such as rice and beans) can provide you with all the essential amino acids. Further, complementary proteins don't need to be eaten within the same meal; you will absorb everything just fine if you eat them within the same day. Ideally, however, you should try to get a balanced mix of both animal and plant proteins, because in addition to the protein, you're also getting vitamins and minerals, and a balance between the two is key.

Where you get it: One cup of plain low-fat yogurt (12 g), 4 ounces of braised lean beef brisket (25 g), 1 cup of cooked chickpeas (14.5 g), 1 ounce of raw cashew nuts (5 g), 1 ounce of nonfat mozzarella cheese (18 g), and 1 large hard-boiled egg (6 g). Most people, expectant moms included, usually have no trouble meeting the daily protein requirement, as protein is found in many different sources, and diets deficient in protein are now quite rare in the industrialized nations. However, not all proteins are created equal, and they are scientifically ranked by their biological value, which reflects how well the protein you consume gets integrated into your and your baby's body. Protein sources that have the highest biological rank include milk, soybeans and soybean milk, eggs, cheese, rice, quinoa, beef, and fish. Another method used to evaluate protein is the Protein Digestibility Corrected Amino Acid Score (PDCAAS), which indicates how well your body can digest the protein. Foods with high rankings on the PDCAAS scale include milk, egg whites, soybeans, beef, chickpeas, black beans, fruits, vegetables, and legumes. As you can see, there is quite a bit of overlap between the PDCAAS and the scientific ranking system, making it easier for you to choose foods that are high in biological value as well as readily digestible.

BE PICKY WITH PROTEINS

It is important to remember that some sources of protein are not recommended during pregnancy, such as high-mercury fish (swordfish, king mackerel, orange roughy, shark, tile fish, big-eye tuna, and marlin), as well as deli and other meats that carry a risk of food pathogens. For more detailed information on foods to avoid, refer to Appendix A.

Calcium

What you need: 1 g per day (1 g per day during breastfeeding)

Why you need it: While your need for calcium remains the same as it was before you got pregnant, it is essential to make sure you're getting enough of it, especially in the second and third trimesters when your baby's bones and teeth are growing and require a continuous calcium supply. Now and until your baby is born, it will need about 30 g of calcium to build strong bones, teeth, a healthy nervous system, heart, and muscles, and to facilitate blood clotting and a normal heart rhythm. The good news is that your body is "cooperating" with you during pregnancy (especially in the second and third trimesters) by significantly increasing your absorption rate of calcium from your diet. However, if your diet does not provide enough calcium and your baby cannot get enough during its development even with your increased absorption rate, baby will "extract" calcium from your own bones (which is where most of your body's calcium is stored), weakening them in the process. Inadequate consumption of calcium also increases the risk for certain pregnancy complications, such as preeclampsia and preterm delivery, whereas adequate calcium intake can help prevent the development of high blood pressure. Statistically, most American women don't consume enough calcium, which is why it's so important to focus on adequate calcium intake at this time.

Studies have also shown that your calcium intake during pregnancy may affect the health and strength of your baby's bones later in life. One study found a link between higher maternal calcium intake and a child's body bone mass (one of the indicators of bone health) at age nine, suggesting the potential effect of calcium intake during pregnancy on the child's bone development later in life. Even though this study looked at children's bones only up to age nine, inadequate maternal calcium intake can potentially have more long-term effects for offspring, such as an increased risk of osteoporosis (reduced bone mineral density, which increases fracture risk).

Where you get it: One cup of plain low-fat yogurt (415 mg), 1 slice of low-fat Swiss cheese (270 mg), 1 cup of raw kale (100 mg), and 1 cup of boiled black-eyed peas (210 mg). Many commonly consumed foods—both dairy and nondairy—are good sources of calcium. Dairy sources include milk, yogurt, natural and processed cheeses, cottage cheese, and ice cream. Great nondairy sources are calcium-fortified orange juice, calcium-set tofu, kale, collard greens, broccoli, sardines, canned salmon with soft bones, dried peas and beans, and roasted almonds. However, even though there are many sources of calcium, a good old glass of milk (as well as plain yogurt) provides the most calcium per single serving (see chart on page 39). Fortified tofu is also a good choice, whereas to get the same amount of calcium from greens (turnip, Chinese cabbage, mustard, kale) and broccoli will require you to consume two to five servings of the food. Last, even though spinach is abundant in calcium, the calcium is not bioavailable, because it contains oxalic acid, which prevents your body from absorbing it (however, spinach is a great source of other nutrients, so you should not avoid it by any means!).

If you think you're falling short or have a hard time getting enough calcium from your diet, talk to your doctor about adding a supplement. A recent review of studies on prenatal calcium supplementation showed a decreased risk of high blood pressure, preeclampsia, severe eclampsia, and preterm birth, and an increase in baby birth weight in those women who took a supplement. However, if your dietary intake is adequate, you likely don't need a supplement,

Got Calcium?

Number of Servings of Different Food Sources That Equal One Serving of Milk

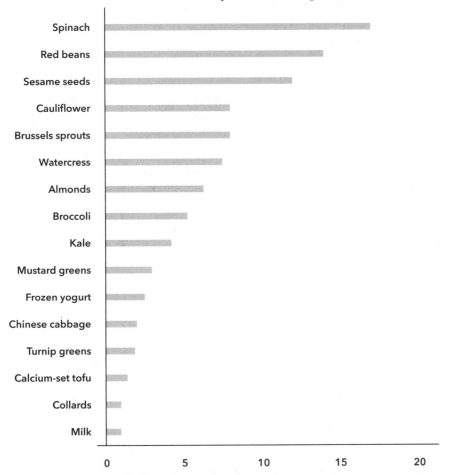

Source: Weaver CM, Proulx WR, Heaney RP. "Choices for achieving dietary calcium within a vegetarian diet." American Journal of Clinical Nutrition 1999;70:543S-548S.

and studies show no effects on the baby's bone mineral mass with calcium supplementation in women who already have adequate calcium intake. In addition, taking in too much calcium can cause constipation (the main side effect of too much calcium) and decrease your absorption of magnesium, so remember that more is not always better.

Fiber

What you need: 28 g per day (29 g per day during breastfeeding)

Why you need it: Constipation is never fun, and it doesn't get any better when you are pregnant! However, there are ways to prevent it. One is to obtain an adequate intake of fiber and water. Throughout your pregnancy, and especially in the second and third trimesters, you should be getting about 28 g of fiber from food sources every day. In addition to being one of the best vanquishers of constipation, fiber is associated with a reduced risk of gestational diabetes, as well as better glucose and insulin regulation throughout pregnancy. It is important to note that there are two types of fiber—soluble and insoluble—and each has different properties. Soluble fiber is fermented in the colon and slows down the passage of food through your digestive system. Insoluble fiber, as the name implies, does not dissolve in water; it is the type of fiber that provides bulk in your colon, helps speed food transit time, and helps you stay regular. In other words, insoluble fiber is more helpful for preventing constipation.

DRINK UP!

When using fiber to combat constipation, don't forget the water—you can think of the two as an inseparable duo, because consuming lots of fiber without drinking plenty of water can actually *cause* constipation.

Where you get it: One cup of cooked split peas (16 g), 1 cup of raw raspberries (8 g), and 1 large apple with skin (5.4 g); or 1 cup of cooked lentils (15.6 g) and 1 cup of cooked artichoke hearts (14.4 g); or 1 cup of cooked black beans (15 g), 1 large raw pear (7 g), and 1 cup of cooked green peas (8.8 g). Many fruits, vegetables, grains, legumes, nuts, and seeds are excellent sources of fiber. If you're eating a well-balanced diet during pregnancy, meeting your fiber needs will likely not be a concern. Pears, prunes, raspberries, strawberries, apples, and mangoes, as well as most veggies (soybeans, artichokes, winter squash, brussels sprouts, leafy greens, broccoli, carrots) and beans (especially navy and pinto), nuts and seeds (pecans, peanuts, walnuts, almonds), cooked oatmeal, wild rice, quinoa, and whole grain breads, cereals, and pastas are all great sources of fiber.

It is in these last three months that your baby puts on the most weight, growing from 2 to about 7.5 pounds. During this time, your baby starts accumulating vitamin and mineral stores (especially iron, calcium, and phosphorus) that will see it through the first six months of life. Most important, your little one's brain development and maturation is fast and furious in the final trimester, making adequate intake of omega-3 fatty acids key in order for your baby's brain to reach its full potential. Because of the speed at which things are happening as well as the number of developmental processes occurring in the last three months, optimal nutrition as well as adequate calories are essential to support your baby's growth, development, and nutrient storage.

Vitamin D

What you need: 15 mcg (600 IUs) per day

Why you need it: Fifteen mcg may not sound like a lot, but this amount of vitamin D can have a major impact during pregnancy. Also known as the "sunshine vitamin" because it can be made by your body upon exposure of the skin to sunlight, vitamin D helps maintain adequate levels of calcium and phosphorus, which are especially important in the third trimester, when your baby's bones and teeth are undergoing the most rapid growth and the majority of the calcium stores (close to 30 g) are deposited. Optimal intake of vitamin D ensures that your baby's bones and teeth develop normally; it has even been linked with long-term health effects, such as a reduced incidence of respiratory tract infections. Vitamin D deficiency, on the other hand, can lead to skeletal abnormalities, reduced birth weight, growth restriction, respiratory infections, preterm birth, "small for gestational age" infants, more fat tissue at birth with potential implications for obesity in later life, and increased odds of needing a C-section. In addition, inadequate intake can increase your risk for preeclampsia, gestational diabetes, and bacterial vaginosis, so make sure you get enough!

Where you get it: Three ounces of cooked sockeye salmon (447 IU), 1 cup of vitamin D–fortified orange juice (150 IU; but check the label, as the amounts can vary quite a bit), and 1 large egg (41 IU; note that only the yolk provides vitamin D). The best sources of vitamin D are animal products such as fatty fish (salmon, canned tuna, canned sardines, catfish), eggs, and D-fortified foods (some common ones are milk, orange juice, margarine, and cereal). However, when choosing the latter foods, be sure to read the label, as not all brands are fortified (some margarines are not fortified), and go for the ones that have added vitamin D to get more of it in your diet. In addition, and especially if you don't live in a place with year-round sunshine, a vitamin D supplement may be beneficial. Speak to your doctor regarding the exact dosage to aim for, because based on current research, an optimal safe dose has not yet been established, even though the overall conclusion based on research is that supplementing is beneficial for increasing the level of maternal serum vitamin D.

SHOULD YOU TAKE A VITAMIN D SUPPLEMENT? ————————

Taking a vitamin D supplement (if it's not in your prenatal vitamin already), especially in the third trimester, may be beneficial because now is the time when your baby is laying down its calcium stores and undergoing rapid bone and teeth growth; vitamin D assists in these processes. While studies have not determined an optimal level of vitamin D supplementation during pregnancy, the 600 IUs/day currently recommended may not be enough. Consult your doctor regarding what's best for you and your baby at this time, while maintaining an intake of at least 600 IUs/day from dietary sources, and if you're falling short of 600 IUs with diet alone (which is especially likely if you're not a fan of fish or are vegetarian or vegan), you should consider adding a supplement to your diet.

Phosphorus

What you need: 700 mg per day (700 mg per day during breastfeeding)

Why you need it: Phosphorus is a mineral that's essential (in addition to calcium and fluoride) for your baby to build strong and healthy bones and teeth; it is also critical for normal blood clotting and heart rhythm, muscle contractions, and nerve signaling. Phosphorus is a key structural component of DNA and RNA molecules and helps you and your baby transport energy in cells.

Where you get it: One cup of plain low-fat yogurt (353 mg), 1 large egg (83 mg), and ½ cup of cooked black beans (281 mg). Any food that contains protein will also contain phosphorus. Generally, if you eat a balanced diet containing enough protein and calcium, you should not be concerned about not getting enough phosphorus. In addition, it is found in smaller quantities in most foods that you eat. Foods that are particularly rich in phosphorus are meats, dairy (yogurt, milk, cheese), fish, poultry, nuts, eggs, and cereals. However, most of the phosphorus in grains is in a form that is poorly absorbed, whereas more than 70 percent of phosphorus in meats is absorbed.

Potassium

What you need: 4.7 g per day (5.1 g during breastfeeding)

Why you need it: Potassium is a key mineral that helps you maintain electrolyte and fluid balance in all your cells. As your blood volume, amniotic fluid, and other body fluids increase dramatically when you're pregnant, adequate intake of potassium is crucial to keep everything in harmony. In addition, potassium is involved in muscle contraction and brain and nerve function.

Where you get it: One large (180 g) sweet potato baked in its skin (855 mg), 1 cup of fresh orange juice (496 mg), 1 cup of baked winter squash (896 mg), 1 cup of cooked lentils (731 mg), 3 ounces of cooked halibut (449 mg), 1 large banana (487 mg), 1½ cups of raw kale (493 mg), and 1 cup of fat-free milk (382 mg). Lots of common foods—mostly unprocessed or only slightly processed foods—contain potassium, such as fresh fruits and vegetables, meat and fish, nuts, seeds, dried fruits, beans, milk and dairy products, and many more. Baked potatoes (sweet and regular potatoes), fruit and vegetable juices (carrot, prune, tomato), coho salmon, plain yogurt, clams, pork, and kidney beans are all great sources of potassium.

Vitamin A

What you need: 770 mcg RAE (retinol activity equivalents) or 2,565 IU per day (1,300 mcg RAE during breastfeeding)

Why you need it: Vitamin A is essential for healthy development of your baby's organs (heart, lungs, brain, kidneys, bones, nerves, and eyes) during the embryonic period, and it is involved in fat metabolism and tissue repair, making it particularly vital as you get closer to your due date. Adequate vitamin A intake and body stores may help your body heal faster after giving birth. Also, vitamin A exists in two forms: preformed vitamin A, or retinol, which is found in animal sources, and provitamin A, or carotenoids (mainly beta-carotene), which are found in plant sources and get converted to retinol in the body. It is important to understand this difference; too much carotene will not harm you, whereas an excess of retinol can lead to liver toxicity and fetal abnormalities. In addition, the average intake of vitamin A in the United States is adequate, as preformed vitamin A is abundant in many animal foods, and numerous plant foods contain lots of provitamin A. Therefore, to avoid the risk of fetal abnormalities and liver toxicity, it is unnecessary and often not recommended to take a vitamin A supplement—especially if the supplement contains the preformed vitamin A.

continued on page 46

Nutritional Needs during Pregnancy

Nutrient	Amount Needed Per Day	Key Function	Food Sources
Calcium	1,000 mg	Crucial for healthy bone and teeth formation, normal blood clotting and heart rhythm, and healthy nervous system	Calcium-set tofu, collard greens, fortified breakfast cereals and fortified orange juice, kale, milk, turnip greens, yogurt
Choline	450 mg	Healthy brain and cell development helps prevent neural tube defects	Broccoli, chicken, eggs, fish, milk, navy beans, nuts, potatoes, quinoa, soybeans, spinach, tofu, wheat germ
EPA and DHA	350 mg EPA, 300 mg DHA	Critical for healthy brain and vision development, associated with better cognitive skills later in life	Anchovies, canned light tuna, catfish, fish oil, fortified eggs, herring, halibut, salmon
Fiber	28 g	Helps prevent constipation, may help prevent gestational diabetes	Beans, fruit, lentils, vegetables, whole grains
Folate/ Folic Acid/ Vitamin B9	600 DFE	Crucial for healthy cell division, helps to prevent neural tube defects	Kidney beans, lentils, kale, spinach
Iron	27 mg	Helps your body make the hemoglobin needed to transport oxygen to all cells	Eggs, fish, fortified cereals, lentils and other legumes, meats, milk, poultry, prune juice, pumpkin seeds, seafood, spinach
Magnesium	350 to 360 mg	Critical component of enzymes, involved in muscle relaxation, may ease leg cramps and prevent preeclampsia and preterm labor	Almonds, baked potato (with skin), bran cereal, brown rice, cashews, halibut, pumpkin seeds, quinoa, salmon, soybeans, spinach, sunflower seeds, tofu, wheat germ
Phosphorus	700 mg	Bone formation, blood clotting, heart rhythm, muscle contractions	Black beans, cereals, cheese, eggs, fish, milk, nuts, poultry, yogurt
Potassium	4.7 g	Electrolyte and fluid balance, brain, nerve and muscle function	Baked sweet potato, banana, kale, lentils, milk, nuts and seeds, orange juice, plain yogurt, winter squash

Nutrient	Amount Needed Per Day	Key Function	Food Sources
Protein	1.1 g per kg of body weight	Contains amino acids, which are the "building blocks" of cells; essential for cell communication and healthy immune system	Beef, black beans, cheese, chickpeas, egg whites, fruits, legumes, milk, quinoa, rice, soybeans, vegetables
Vitamin A	770 mcg RAE or 2,565 IU	Healthy organ development, tissue repair, wound healing	Cantaloupe, carrots, cheese, eggs, kale, oatmeal, spinach, sweet potato
Vitamin B6	1.9 mg	Helps metabolize carbohydrate, protein, and fat; helps make new red blood cells and is needed for healthy brain development; may help prevent nausea	Avocado, baked potato, banana, brown rice, chicken, chickpeas, pork loin, prune juice, salmon, spinach
Vitamin B12	2.6 mcg	Brain and nervous system development, DNA synthesis, fatty acid and protein synthesis, blood formation; may help prevent neural tube defects	Beef, cod, cheese, eggs milk, salmon
Vitamin C	85 mg	Wound healing, tissue repair, healthy skin maintenance, collagen synthesis, bone development	Bell peppers (yellow, green, red), broccoli, brussels sprouts, guava, kiwifruit, mango, oranges, papaya, sweet potato
Vitamin D	15 mcg (600 IU)	Critical for healthy bone and teeth development	Egg yolks, fatty fish (salmon, trout), fortified milk and orange juice
Vitamin K	90 mcg	Essential for normal blood clotting	Brussels sprouts, cabbage, collards, kale, mustard greens, spinach
Zinc	11 mg	Essential mineral for healthy cell division, DNA and protein synthesis, supports a healthy immune system	Alaskan king crab, collard greens, garbanzo and kidney beans, ground beef, milk, pumpkin seeds, tofu, turkey, whole grains

Where you get it: Half cup of raw kale (168 RAE), 3 ounces of baby carrots (586 RAE), and 1 large hard-boiled egg (74 RAE) or ½ cup (100 g) of sweet potato baked in the skin (961 RAE). Both types of vitamin A are abundant in commonly eaten foods, such as carrots, eggs, kale, oatmeal, cantaloupe, spinach, sweet potato, cheese, and many others. You don't have to worry about your carotenoid intake (and some veggies, such as sweet potato, can be very high in it), but do limit your intake of animal foods that have lots of the preformed vitamin A, such as liver, to prevent any detrimental consequences of taking in too much vitamin A. I doubt that liver will be high on your list of most craved foods, but if it is, I would advise avoiding liver completely during pregnancy, as its vitamin A concentration is so high that eating even a couple of bites can put you way over your daily recommendation for vitamin A intake (and can even exceed the safe upper limit). Finally, know that retinol and beta-carotene are not equal in terms of the potency of vitamin A—it takes twelve times more beta-carotene (provitamin A) to equal 1 mcg of retinol, or preformed vitamin A.

Vitamin C

What you need: 85 mg per day (120 mg during breastfeeding)

Why you need it: Vitamin C, or ascorbic acid, is an antioxidant that protects your cells and your baby's cells from oxidative damage; helps your body fight infections, heal wounds, and repair tissues; and is involved in collagen synthesis, thus helping to maintain healthy skin. Collagen isn't just for filling wrinkles; in fact, it is crucial for your developing baby, as collagen is a structural component of connective tissues such as tendons, cartilage, blood vessels, bone matrix, and corneas, making adequate vitamin C intake essential for healthy growth and development.

Where you get it: One glass of orange juice (124 mg), or 1 cup of strawberries (85 mg), or 2 cups of chopped raw collards (25 mg) and 1 kiwifruit (64 mg), or 1 small raw red bell pepper (95 mg). Many fresh fruits and vegetables contain vitamin C, especially citrus fruits and leafy greens; these include oranges, broccoli, guava, papaya, bell peppers (yellow, green, red), sweet potato, mango, brussels sprouts, and many others. Keep in mind that vitamin C is easily lost during cooking, so raw fruits and veggies are your best bet.

Vitamin K

What you need: 90 mcg per day (same amount during breastfeeding)

Why you need it: Vitamin K is essential for normal blood clotting, and adequate stores become increasingly important as you're nearing your due date because lots of blood is lost at delivery (both vaginal and Cesarean), and adequate intake will improve optimal blood clotting.

Where you get it: One cup of raw spinach (145 mcg), ½ cup of chopped kale (236 mcg), or 1 cup of broccoli (220 mcg). Leafy greens are the main source of vitamin K: collards, spinach, kale, cabbage, mustard greens, Swiss chard, brussels sprouts, and others are all excellent sources of the vitamin.

* * *

Whew! That was a lot of information, but now I bet you know more than you ever thought you would about nutrition in pregnancy. Now that we have covered the key nutrients for a healthy pregnancy and baby, *why* they are key, and *where* you can find them, we can move on to Part II of the book. The three chapters in Part II delve into the three trimesters of pregnancy, week by week, so you can see how your baby is developing and learn how you can support your baby's growth through good nutrition.

This certainly doesn't mean that you need to eat *all* of the foods discussed here or in the next section every day. Remember that most foods you consume contain multiple nutrients. For example, cooked lentils contain folate, iron, fiber, phosphorus, protein, B vitamins (B1, B5, and B6, to be exact), potassium, zinc, manganese (which we haven't discussed, but is important in developing baby's bones and cartilage), and copper (also not discussed—this mineral, found in all plant and animal tissues, is essential to forming red blood cells), helping you get part of your daily dose of all of these nutrients. Your goal is to try to eat foods that are healthy, wholesome, and contain nutrients that we know will be beneficial to you and your baby. Plus, the week-by-week guide will help make eating healthy manageable, and maybe even fun, because you will understand how the great food you are eating is helping your little one develop and grow up strong!

PART II

What to Eat during the Stages of Pregnancy— A Week-by-Week Guide

CHAPTER 4

The First Trimester

The first three months of your pregnancy, otherwise known as the first trimester, are especially important, as the cells in your baby's body are rapidly growing and differentiating, eventually forming the skeletal system and the various organs and organ systems, such as the nervous and cardiovascular systems. Throughout your pregnancy, there are certain periods, called "critical windows," when particular organs or tissues develop. During these periods, proper nutrition is especially important, as risk for damage to these organs or tissues is increased.

In this chapter I will discuss each of the critical windows that take place during the first trimester and provide a week-by-week guide to the development of your baby as well as a description of foods that you can focus on each week to promote this development.

But first, let's talk about one of the less-pleasant aspects of pregnancy for some expectant mothers: morning sickness.

Morning Sickness and How to Relieve It with Food

Whoever coined the term "morning sickness" was clearly never pregnant, because unfortunately you can have it morning, noon, and night! Morning sickness is the feeling of nausea, with or without vomiting, that many women experience while pregnant. The specific causes of morning sickness are debated and not fully understood, although hormones, psychological factors, and slowed digestion may play a role.

Most pregnant women experience some morning sickness in the early months. In fact, a recent study found that almost 70 percent of pregnant women in the United States suffer from some form of it. Often starting between weeks 4 and 6 and peaking between weeks 8 and 12, nausea and vomiting may be quite problematic for some women. A minority (about 1.2 percent) may experience a severe form of morning sickness, called *hyperemesis gravidarum,* when vomiting occurs every day and can lead to a loss of more than 5 percent of prepregnancy body weight. Kate Middleton's battle with this type of severe morning sickness during her pregnancies in 2012 and 2014 was highly publicized. This more severe form of morning sickness may cause a woman to become nutrient deficient and dehydrated (not to mention make her feel awful), which in turn may harm the baby, causing a low birth weight or preterm delivery. Fortunately, there is a light at the end of the tunnel: though about one in five women may continue to experience symptoms beyond the 20th week, for most, symptoms of morning sickness tend to improve by week 16.

If you are experiencing morning sickness, you know how difficult it can be to constantly feel like you're about to throw up and to not be able to function as you did just a few weeks ago. But most important, you may be concerned about your baby. Is it getting enough nutrients if you're constantly nauseous and vomiting and having trouble eating? How can you relieve your nausea and keep food down? Fortunately, there are a few natural remedies you can try.

TRIGGERS OF MORNING SICKNESS

If you've already experienced nausea or vomiting, think about the situation or environment that you were in when the symptoms began, and try to identify what might have triggered that reaction. There are a few factors that can bring on nausea, such as being in a crowded or stuffy room; the smell of certain foods, perfumes or colognes, smoke, and other chemicals; and environmental conditions, such as heat, humidity, or being surrounded by noise. If you notice that any of these (or other) factors tend to make you nauseous, try to avoid them. In addition, try to avoid food smells until the moment you start eating, as they can trigger nausea. It may also be helpful to consider whether any food textures might have triggered your nausea in the past so you can avoid them in the future. Also try to avoid sudden movements, such as getting out of bed too fast. Last, if you're taking an iron supplement (or if iron is part of your prenatal vitamin), talk to your doctor about your iron level and whether it might be beneficial to go off of it until your symptoms improve, as iron supplements can cause nausea and vomiting.

Change Up Your Eating Pattern

Try to eat a number of small meals (aim for about six per day) slowly instead of larger meals, because a full stomach can trigger nausea and vomiting. Similarly, an empty stomach can make you feel sick, so try not to go too long between meals. It can be helpful to keep a snack handy. Speaking of which, having a snack, such as a banana or crackers, even *before* getting out of bed may also help.

Become a Food Detective

Try to figure out which foods you can tolerate without getting nauseous. If you find that hot foods trigger nausea, go with cold foods instead, as their smell is not as intense so they may be easier to handle. Avoid greasy or fried foods, as they can trigger nausea from the smell as well as cause it after eating, because fats are more difficult to digest than carbohydrates or proteins. Try to go for low-fat, protein-rich foods, such as eggs, lean meat, or boiled beans, and try to take in more liquids than solids. Additionally, try salty liquids, such as sports drinks with electrolytes, in small volumes (preferably half an hour before or after you eat so that you avoid having a full stomach). Choosing cold, carbonated, and slightly sour liquids may also help, so if you start feeling nauseous, try sipping on a cool, carbonated beverage, such as ginger ale or lemonade (it may be helpful to always keep a few cans in the fridge). Eliminating coffee, spicy and smelly, high-fat, very sweet, or very sour foods and choosing more bland, low-fat, salty, or dry foods, such as crackers, pretzels, or toast, may also help alleviate symptoms of morning sickness.

The Power of Ginger

Ginger is the only nondrug intervention for treating nausea and vomiting recommended by the American Congress of Obstetrics and Gynecology. It is thought to help improve symptoms by stimulating your digestive tract motility and the flow of saliva, bile, and gastric secretions. Several studies have shown that women reported reduced nausea (but, unfortunately, not reduced vomiting) when given ginger compared to a placebo. Overall, ginger has been recognized as safe for use during pregnancy and effective in alleviating nausea; it is recommended if you're experiencing morning sickness. No detrimental consequences to the mother or the baby have been noted with ginger use in small quantities. However, it is important to note that the maximum safe dose of ginger, as well as ginger's interactions with other herbs, is unknown. Thus you should avoid consuming it in high doses or in combination with herbs; ideally, stick to ginger tea or other forms of ginger that provide small amounts.

Make Sure You Are Getting Enough Vitamin B6

In addition to the many benefits of vitamin B6 mentioned in the last chapter, this vitamin has also been shown to be effective in alleviating the nausea associated with morning sickness and may even be as effective in treating nausea as ginger. Make sure you get enough B6 in your diet (1.9 mg per day), and if you're concerned that you're not getting the required amount, or if you want to try it as a nausea-alleviating agent, talk to your doctor about adding a vitamin B6 supplement (if you're taking a prenatal vitamin, be sure to check the package, as B6 may already be in there).

WHAT ABOUT ACUPRESSURE BANDS?

These are bands worn on your wrists with small buttons that lightly press on a specific point and may alleviate symptoms of nausea and vomiting. The research on the effectiveness of these bands has been mixed, but some studies show that they may help relieve the symptoms of morning sickness. While other studies suggest that ginger may be more effective than acupressure, acupressure is still better at reducing nausea than no intervention at all. Because there is no harm associated with using acupressure bands, at the very least it doesn't hurt to give them a shot! They may be effective for you, whether due to a real benefit of the band pressing on a particular point or a placebo effect. If it works, who cares, right?

If you are experiencing morning sickness—whether mild, moderate, or severe—talk to your doctor and start by trying the natural interventions described here as your first line of defense. If these approaches don't help, or if you have a severe form of morning sickness, your doctor may consider prescribing a medication. There are safe medications for use in pregnancy that have proven to be effective in alleviating both nausea and vomiting.

Your First Trimester Week by Week

Now that we've tackled the least fun aspect of early pregnancy, let's travel through the first trimester week by week to see how your baby is growing and developing during the first 12 weeks of life in the womb. For each week, I will briefly describe the key developmental processes that are occurring and suggest a "food of the week," which you can incorporate into different dishes while continuing to eat a balanced diet. I have also listed some recipes for each week that you might try, as well as other suggestions for ways to easily incorporate the food of the week into your diet.

HOW OLD IS MY BABY?

Your baby's age while in the womb can be counted in two ways: by conceptional age or gestational age. Conceptional age is based on the day your baby was conceived, while gestational age is based on the first day of your last menstrual period. Both methods are a bit tricky. Conceptional age may seem like the logical way of counting your baby's age, but many women don't know exactly when they got pregnant. Even if you've been tracking things like a detective, you still may have no clue when your egg was fertilized, since a few days can pass between the time of intercourse and fertilization. Sperm need some time to reach their destination and do their job. Gestational age, on the other hand, starts counting your baby's "age" before it actually exists; it considers your last period and the days before you conceived as the beginning of pregnancy, which is also a bit confusing. Here are nice rules of thumb for calculating either: If you know the exact date of conception, add two weeks and you'll get gestational age. If you know the first day of your last period, subtract two weeks and you'll get conceptional age. To make it easier to understand, I will use conceptional age when describing the different stages of pregnancy and include the gestational age in parentheses next to each week's heading.

Week 1

(Gestational Week 3)

This is the germinal stage: fertilization and implantation.

What's Happening?

The first week is when fertilization occurs, meaning that your egg and your partner's sperm cell combine to produce a zygote with forty-six chromosomes. Your baby's sex is defined at the moment of conception, depending on whether it receives an X (female) or a Y (male) chromosome from the father. The zygote travels to your uterus, rapidly dividing on its way (it is now a ball of cells called a blastocyst). Around day 7 following fertilization, the zygote implants in the lining of your uterus and begins to receive nutrients from your body.

It may be helpful to note that at this stage, the fertilized egg is thought to be not very susceptible to toxic agents, such as drugs or alcohol. This is not meant to be a green light to hit happy hour; if the trauma from a toxin is severe enough, it can cause a termination of the pregnancy, even though you may not even know you are pregnant at this time and may not notice anything. If the baby survives, however, toxins are not thought to cause abnormalities this early on. So if you did have a glass (or two) of wine during this week (when most women don't even know they are pregnant), don't sweat it.

Food of the Week: Lentils

Early on in pregnancy, folate is key, and lentils are simply packed with it. In addition, they're a good source of iron to start building up your stores from the very beginning. Lentils also contain fiber, phosphorus, protein, vitamin B6, potassium, zinc, and copper, among other nutrients. A cup of cooked lentils (about 200 g) contains more than half of your daily folate requirement (about 360 mcg; you need 600 per day). Simple to prepare and easy to digest, lentils are wonderful in soup, salad, or a side dish.

Easy Seasoned Lentils

SERVES 2

For a protein- and fiber-rich vegetarian entrée, try these lentils spooned over baked potatoes or sweet potatoes. Double the recipe for excellent leftovers, which can be used to fill wraps or whole wheat pitas. Leftovers also freeze well for make-ahead meals.

1¾ cups water
½ cup brown lentils
1 carrot, chopped
½ cup chopped tomatoes, fresh or canned and drained
1 cup chopped celery
¼ teaspoon each salt, onion powder, garlic powder, turmeric, and cinnamon
1 teaspoon hot sauce
1 teaspoon extra-virgin olive oil

Bring the water to a boil, then add the lentils, carrot, tomatoes, and celery and reduce the heat to low. Cover and simmer for 30 minutes.

Uncover and add the salt, onion powder, garlic powder, turmeric, cinnamon, hot sauce, and oil. Stir and cook until the liquid is absorbed, about 5 minutes. Serve warm.

Week 2

(Gestational Week 4)

This is when cells begin to differentiate.

What's Happening?

Starting in week 2, the zygote is already implanted in your uterus and is actively developing, even though it's so tiny that it would still not be visible to the naked eye. It is receiving oxygen and some nutrients from you directly, but the placenta is starting to form, preparing the nutrient supply line for your baby as it grows bigger. The cells of the embryo are rapidly differentiating, meaning that they are getting ready to become specialized cells to form the many different organs and organ systems that will make up your baby's body.

Just like in the first week, in the second week post-conception, the embryo is still not very susceptible to the mother's lifestyle choices such as drinking, smoking, or inadequate nutrition. Again, not a green light to party all night, but don't worry too much if you have imbibed!

Food of the Week: Spinach

Whether raw or cooked, spinach is another excellent source of folate, which is more essential early on than at any other point in pregnancy. Three cups of raw spinach (about 90 g) will provide you with roughly a third of the folate you need per day, whereas a cup of boiled spinach (without salt) contains almost half (260 DFEs). Spinach is also rich in potassium, iron, vitamin A, phosphorus, and magnesium. An easy way to get your spinach is raw in a salad or cooked as a side dish. In addition to the recipe below, also check out the Arugula Salad with Turkey, Avocado, and Dried Cranberries (page 65) and the Rotisserie Chicken with Apricot Quinoa over Spinach (page 89).

Cauliflower, Celery, and Spinach Soup

MAKES 8 CUPS

This creamy vegetable soup is a delicious low-calorie first course with folate, fiber, and minerals, a great way to start your meal. It's also a delicious lunch alongside a grilled cheese or turkey sandwich.

1 head cauliflower, chopped
8 ribs celery
4 cups chicken or vegetable broth
¼ cup light cream cheese
1 bunch spinach, roughly chopped (or a 5-ounce bag of baby spinach)
½ teaspoon onion powder
⅛ teaspoon freshly ground black pepper

Combine the cauliflower, celery, and broth in a saucepan. Bring to a boil over high heat, then reduce the heat to medium-low and simmer for 10 minutes.

Transfer about half of the mixture to a blender and add the cream cheese. Cover and process until smooth. (If your blender lid has a central cap that can be removed, remove it and drape a dishtowel over the top so steam can escape while processing.) Return the mixture to the pot, add the spinach, onion powder, and pepper, and simmer for 5 minutes more. Serve hot.

Week 3

(Gestational Week 5)

This is when the embryonic period begins.

What's Happening?

Your baby is now beginning what is called the embryonic period, which will continue until the end of week 8 and is marked by rapid development of the key organs and organ systems. During week 3, the cells of the embryo form into three distinct layers that give rise to the various tissues and organs of your baby's body. Also during this time, some of the most essential organs start to form, including the heart, the spinal cord, the digestive tract, and the lungs.

With week 3 begins the time when your baby is highly susceptible to environmental toxins and harmful agents, as well as inadequate maternal nutrition. Alcohol use during this time can lead to spontaneous abortion or severe fetal abnormalities, such as fetal alcohol syndrome.

Just because developmental problems can occur in response to toxins during this time doesn't mean that they *will*. Many women don't even know that they are pregnant at this point, as menstrual cycles can vary depending on several factors, including stress. Also, if you weren't paying attention to your cycle, or maybe not necessarily trying to get pregnant, then you might not realize you are late this week. Not to worry! A recent study in Ireland looked at alcohol consumption in women throughout their pregnancy and found no significant differences in preterm birth, low birth weight, or growth restriction between women who consumed some alcohol during the first trimester and those who didn't. In addition, the researchers did not find any significant differences in the same outcomes when women consumed alcohol in the third trimester. The reported alcohol consumption in women who drank alcohol was moderate, with the majority consuming 5 units of alcohol or less per week. To put this into perspective, a 175-mL glass of 12-percent alcohol red wine is approximately 2 units.

Food of the Week: Asparagus

A cup of cooked asparagus (180 g) has about half of the daily folate you need (270 DFEs) and contains other key nutrients, such as potassium, phosphorus, vitamins A, C, and K, and others. Fresh asparagus is ideal, but if your grocery store does not always carry it (due to its short growing season), then use frozen or canned asparagus.

In addition to the following recipe, there are several easy ways to get more asparagus into your diet.

- Chop it up and toss it into a pan with scrambled eggs.

- Sauté whole stalks in a little olive oil with a sprinkle of bread crumbs on top. The bread crumbs give great texture!

- Serve it with other veggies! Add chopped asparagus to your raw veggie plate. It is great for dipping and not at all messy to handle.

- Make it an add-in to just about any dish. Asparagus doesn't have to be the star of the meal. You can have some on hand and add it to salads and pasta and grain dishes. It will add color and make the shape and texture of your meal unique.

Asparagus with Lemon Zest and Paprika

SERVES 4

With only three ingredients, this low-calorie, low-sodium recipe couldn't be easier or more healthful!

1 pound asparagus, ends trimmed
Zest from 1 lemon
Paprika

Place the asparagus in a ceramic or glass casserole dish with a lid. Add 2 tablespoons of water to the dish, cover, and microwave for 5 minutes. Stir and check for doneness. (If desired, cook 1 or 2 additional minutes.) Drain the water from the dish and pat the asparagus with a paper towel to absorb any excess moisture. Sprinkle evenly with the lemon zest and paprika and serve.

GROW YOUR OWN

One fun thing you can do is grow your own asparagus. Even if you don't have a green thumb, they are easy to grow, and the best part is that they are perennials, which means they come back every year! When I was pregnant with my daughter, I planted some in our garden (ask for "asparagus crowns" at your garden center). Just like a baby, they take a few years to mature! The first year they are skinny twigs that you can't really eat, but by years 3 and 4 (when your little one is curious and can help you garden), the edible new shoots are bigger and can be harvested. Planting your asparagus bed is a fun and easy activity you can do with your new baby before it even arrives!

Week 4

(Gestational Week 6)

Your baby is now the size of a grain of rice and has a heartbeat.

What's Happening?

Your baby's brain, heart, lungs, muscle, liver, pancreas, jaws, eyes, nose, palate, central nervous system, and many other body parts are now developing at a fast pace. Most importantly and excitingly, your baby now has a beating heart that is pumping blood through its still super-tiny body and delivering nutrients to the key developing tissues. The heart and the cardiovascular system are some of the first organs and systems to form and function in the embryo, because it cannot continue to get all the nutrients and oxygen into its little body via simple diffusion and needs a more efficient way to get its supplies. By the end of week 4, the neural tube fully closes. A functional fetal-placental circulation system is now established, and all organs are now prepared for growth!

Week 4 is part of a very sensitive embryonic developmental period, and the risks remain high for all of the major structural abnormalities: central nervous system, heart, limbs, eyes, ears, and others. Alcohol and drugs continue to pose a high risk for fetal abnormalities, and nutritional deficiencies can directly affect the organs developing at this time. Also noteworthy: this is the last week when the embryo is still highly sensitive to folate deficiency, as the neural tube is completing its closure. However, folate continues to be important beyond this point, as it is needed for other developmental processes.

Food of the Week: Beets

Beets are another excellent source of folate (1 cup of beets supplies a quarter of the daily folate you need), potassium, phosphorus, and magnesium. A great way to get your beets is in smoothies—you can toss some apples, carrots, and celery into the mix, blend them together, and voilà—a delicious and nutritious drink! Just remember to thoroughly scrub and wash the beets under running water with a veggie brush to get rid of all the dirt as well as potential bacteria that may be lurking on its rough surface before you cook them. If you consume raw beets, you should peel the skin off.

Roasted or Raw Beet Salad

SERVES 2

This salad is incredibly simple to make and tastes delicious whether you leave the beets raw or choose to roast them. (Roasting makes them sweeter and softer.) Add a squeeze of lemon and chopped apple or pear for a fruity twist. To make a well-rounded meal, top with chicken or goat cheese, or add some walnuts or pumpkin seeds for a complementary crunch.

1 beet (the size of a baseball), scrubbed
1 to 2 tablespoons extra-virgin olive oil, more if you like
2 cups finely chopped kale, tough stems removed

Salt and freshly ground black pepper

Optional toppings: Squeeze of lemon, chopped apple or pear, shredded or cubed cooked chicken, goat cheese, walnuts, or roasted pumpkin seeds

If you plan to use the beets raw, be sure to peel off the skin (this is optional if you're roasting them) and, using a spiral slicer, mandoline, or julienne peeler, cut the beet into long, thin noodles. If roasting the beets, preheat the oven to 400°F. Toss the beets with 1 tablespoon of the olive oil and place on a baking sheet. Cook for 10 to 15 minutes until slightly tender (soft but not mushy, like al dente pasta).

Combine the beets and kale in a large bowl and toss to coat the kale with 1 tablespoon of the oil. Add salt and pepper to taste, and serve with additional toppings of your choice.

Week 5

(Gestational Week 7)

In your growing baby, every essential organ has begun to form.

What's Happening?

Your baby is growing fast yet is still very tiny (only about ¼ centimeter) and looks more like a tadpole than a little human being. By now, almost every part of its body has started to form: eyelids, ears, mouth, tongue, heart, lung, muscle, liver, pancreas, brain, and others. All of these will continue to develop, but the foundation for their development has been laid down. Additionally, the buds that will develop into arms and legs are sprouting.

Food of the Week: Wild Salmon

Rich in healthy mono- and polyunsaturated fatty acids, as well as protein, vitamin B12, niacin, potassium, phosphorus, and zinc, wild salmon is an excellent source of nutrients for your baby in this phase of speedy development. Omega-3 fatty acids, in which wild salmon is particularly rich (farmed salmon also contains omega-3s, though less than the wild varieties), are crucial for healthy brain development, which is now occurring and will continue until birth and beyond. In addition to the recipe below, check out the Mom-Safe Sushi Bowl (page 107).

Maple-Soy Glazed Salmon

SERVES 2

Oily fish such as salmon and trout are the richest food sources of long-chain omega-3 fatty acids, a key nutrient for healthy pregnancy. This easy glazed salmon has a perfect blend of sweet and salty flavor. Serve alongside asparagus and baked potatoes for restaurant-quality fare at home.

1 pound wild salmon or trout
2 teaspoons maple syrup
2 teaspoons soy sauce
Pinch of hot pepper flakes (optional)

Preheat the oven to 425°F. Line a baking sheet with foil and place the fish on it, skin-side down. Bake for 10 to 15 minutes, until the flesh flakes easily with a fork.

While the fish is cooking, combine the syrup and soy sauce in a small pot and bring to a boil over medium heat. Boil for 60 seconds, then turn off heat. The mixture will thicken into a syrup-consistency glaze.

When the fish is done, pour the glaze over it, spreading evenly with a spatula. Sprinkle with hot pepper flakes and serve immediately.

Week 6

(Gestational Week 8)

Your baby is the size of a jelly bean.

What's Happening?

Your baby continues to be hard at work developing its tissues, organs, and body parts. Your baby's kidneys are now forming; blood cells are being produced at high rates by the spleen and liver, and some are being made by the bones. The baby's heart has separated into two chambers (it will separate into all four later on) and is now beating at 150 beats per minute—twice as fast as your own!

Food of the Week: Bananas

Bananas are an excellent source of potassium and are also high in carbohydrates, with some magnesium, phosphorus, and vitamin C. It may be a good idea to eat one first thing in the morning, as it could help prevent or reduce any nausea that you may be experiencing. Week 6 is the time when the dreaded morning sickness usually kicks in, and you may be finding it difficult to eat or keep food down. You may be experiencing a lack of appetite or even feel repelled by the mere thought of food. If that's the case, check out the morning sickness relief tips on page 50, and if things are too difficult to manage on your own, be sure to speak with your doctor. In addition to the recipe below, check out the Frozen Banana–Chocolate–Peanut Butter Bites (page 88). The following simple recipe may be one of the easier foods to keep down at this time.

Banana and Almond Butter Wrap

SERVES 1

Only have a minute to make lunch? Don't feel like hanging out in the kitchen? Whip up this satisfying wrap in no time flat—this nutritious meal may be the easiest thing you do all day.

2 tablespoons unsalted almond butter
1 whole wheat tortilla
1 banana, peeled and cut in half lengthwise
Cinnamon

Spread the almond butter down the center of the tortilla. Place the two banana halves on top of the almond butter, sprinkle lightly with cinnamon, and roll up the tortilla. Eat it right away or warm it in the microwave for about 20 seconds first.

Week 7

(Gestational Week 9)

Your baby is now about ½ inch long.

What's Happening?

In addition to all of the body parts and organs that are already rapidly developing, your baby's teeth and palate are starting to form. Now and in the next few weeks, as your baby's body continues to grow and develop, every day each organ becomes more specialized and complicated. This week is a peak time for morning sickness for many women; if this is true for you, you may need to put in a lot of extra effort to take in the proper nutrients and keep them down.

Food of the Week: Sweet Potato

High in carbohydrates, potassium, iron, magnesium, phosphorus, and vitamins A, C, and K, sweet potatoes are a great source of nutrients at this time. In addition, because they contain plenty of carbohydrates and vitamin B6, sweet potatoes may be especially beneficial if you're experiencing nausea and vomiting. Baking it with the skin on is one of the best choices, although any form is good. Nutrient-packed and delicious, the following recipe not only provides you with the vitamins and minerals you need but may even help with the morning sickness (cinnamon is known for alleviating nausea in pregnancy). Though baking is involved, the preparation is very easy. However, if you don't feel like adding cinnamon or think that it may trigger your nausea (every woman is different, and what helps some with nausea may actually trigger it in others), you can easily omit it and enjoy a simple, plain baked sweet potato.

Cinnamon Baked Sweet Potato Wedges

SERVES 2

Baked sweet potato wedges are a tasty alternative to sweet potato fries. Adding a dash of cinnamon perks up the flavor, and if you like them with a little kick, add a sprinkle of cayenne pepper too.

1 sweet potato or yam (½ pound)
2 teaspoons extra-virgin olive oil
Salt
Cinnamon
Cayenne pepper (optional)

Preheat the oven to 350°F and line a baking sheet with foil. Wash the sweet potato and cut it in half lengthwise, then slice each half into 4 thin wedges for 8 total. If any wedges are thicker than 1 inch at the widest part, slice those in half again.

Place the sweet potatoes in a mixing bowl and add the oil. Toss to coat. Spread the sweet potatoes on the baking sheet, leaving room between them, and sprinkle lightly with salt, cinnamon, and cayenne to taste.

Bake for 45 minutes, or until tender with crisp edges. Serve hot or warm.

Week 8

(Gestational Week 10)

This week your baby's embryonic period ends; from this point on, it is a fetus.

What's Happening?

Week 8 is an important one, because by the end of it, your baby will have completed the embryonic development period: all of its major body systems will have formed. All of these will continue to grow and develop throughout the rest of the pregnancy: fingers and toes, brain (250,000 neurons are produced per minute!), heart, lungs, muscle, liver, pancreas, kidney, and blood vessels, to list just a few. Interestingly, during this time your baby's taste buds are forming on its little tongue, and the eyelids are now covering a larger area of the eyes.

Food of the Week: Turkey

Roasted turkey without the skin is a great source of iron, phosphorus, potassium, zinc, niacin, and lean protein—and all of these nutrients are needed to support your baby's development at this time. If you're having a hard time keeping food down, try eating the turkey cold, such as in a salad like the following recipe, as it will be close to odorless and bland tasting, making it easier to eat. This recipe is delicious and not overwhelming flavor-wise—try it for a wholesome, light, and balanced meal. In addition to the recipe below, check out Savory Roasted Chicken Breasts with Whole Grain Mustard (page 83), Two-Pepper Turkey and Havarti Sandwich with Radish Salad (page 91), and Turkey-Apple Burgers with Cheddar (page 99).

Arugula Salad with Turkey, Avocado, and Dried Cranberries

SERVES 2

Peppery arugula makes a delicious salad base and is high in magnesium, vitamin A, and folate. The creamy avocado and sweet cranberries round out the flavors of this colorful, nutrient-packed salad.

6 ounces baby arugula (or baby spinach)
8 ounces cooked turkey breast
⅔ avocado, cubed

4 tablespoons dried cranberries
1½ cups cherry tomatoes, halved
2 to 4 tablespoons vinaigrette dressing of your choice

Combine the arugula, turkey, avocado, cranberries, tomatoes, and dressing in a large mixing bowl and toss gently to coat. Divide the salad between two plates and serve.

Week 9

(Gestational Week 11)

The fetal period begins—let's build some muscle!

What's Happening?

Week 9 is a very exciting one, as your baby has now begun what is known as the fetal period, which will last until birth. Most of the major organs (heart, lungs, liver, pancreas, kidneys, blood vessels, brain), which have been developing throughout, are continuing to grow, and now your baby is actively building its muscles. In addition, its kidneys have just started to do their job, and urine formation begins between weeks 9 and 12. Your baby will start discharging urine into the amniotic fluid, which will then be transferred to your circulation, processed, and expelled from your body. At the end of this week, your baby is about 2.2 centimeters long—still short of an inch, but slowly getting there!

Food of the Week: Pumpkin Seeds

Pumpkin seeds are one of the best sources of nonanimal iron and are also rich in protein, magnesium, phosphorus, potassium, zinc, niacin, vitamin K, and mono- and polyunsaturated fatty acids. In their raw (unroasted, unsalted) form, pumpkin seeds are also essentially odorless, making them easier to eat if you're experiencing morning sickness. Pumpkin seeds can be an excellent snack between meals, or you can sprinkle them on a salad, adding many important nutrients to your diet without much effort. In addition to the recipe below, check out the Roasted or Raw Beet Salad (page 60).

Harvest Oatmeal with Pumpkin Seeds

SERVES 2

Rich in whole grains, vitamin A, fiber, and calcium, this warm bowl of fall-flavored goodness is tasty any day of the year. It's a great way to use up canned pumpkin from another recipe, or leftover cranberry sauce from your holiday feast. Just freeze pumpkin and cranberry sauce in ice-cube trays, then pop the cubes into a resealable plastic bag for longer storage.

1 cup quick-cooking ("baby") oats
3 cups skim, 1%, or almond milk
⅔ cup canned pumpkin puree
½ cup cranberry sauce (homemade or canned)
1 teaspoon pumpkin pie spice
¼ teaspoon salt
2 tablespoons roasted pumpkin seeds

Combine all of the ingredients (except the pumpkin seeds) in a small pot and cook over medium heat until bubbling. Reduce the heat to low and cook, stirring, for 1 minute. Pour into a bowl and sprinkle with the pumpkin seeds.

Week 10

(Gestational Week 12)

Let's get physical: your baby is starting to stretch and kick.

What's Happening?

During this time, as your baby's main organs continue to grow, baby is also hard at work building bones and cartilage. This week, the fingernails also start to appear, and the eyelids are even better formed (though they are still fused shut). Now that all of the main organs are beginning to work, your baby can swallow amniotic fluid. The baby's heart has divided into all four chambers and is working hard to pump blood as well as deliver oxygen and nutrients throughout its growing body. Perhaps most exciting, your baby is also starting to stretch and kick—though you won't feel this for another month or two. Week 10 is also an important one if the baby is a boy, as his testes now start to produce testosterone!

Food of the Week: Eggs

As discussed in more detail in Appendix A (along with other tips about foods to avoid), you should consume only eggs that are thoroughly cooked to kill any potential salmonella. Properly cooked eggs, however, are an excellent food, particularly at this time. Eggs are rich in protein, iron, phosphorus, zinc, and vitamins A and D, as well as monounsaturated fatty acids. Two hard-boiled eggs with one or two slices of whole wheat toast can be a perfect breakfast. If you're experiencing nausea or vomiting, try eating the hard-boiled eggs cold, as they will have next to no odor and thus may be easier to eat and keep down. In addition to the recipes below, check out Turkey-Apple Burgers with Cheddar (page 99); Anchovy, Parsley, and Parmesan Cheese Quiche (page 112); and Stuffed Portobello Caps with Wild Rice, Cherries, and Pecans (page 114).

Egg, Toast, and Melon Plate

SERVES 2

This meal is gentle on the stomach and gives you steady energy that will take you through a challenging morning. Try this for a low-odor, easy-to-digest meal that provides a balance of protein, carbohydrates, and fat, with a replenishing dose of potassium. If desired, add a sprinkle of salt to the eggs.

4 eggs
4 slices whole grain bread
2 cups cut melon (honeydew or cantaloupe)

Place the eggs in a single layer in the bottom of a saucepan and add enough cold water to cover by at least an inch. Bring to a boil, then reduce the heat to low and simmer for 12 minutes. Drain, keeping the eggs in the pot, and immediately refill the pot with cold water (this shock makes them easier to peel). Let sit for a minute before draining again. The eggs will keep in the refrigerator for up to a week.

Peel and slice the eggs and toast the bread. Serve the eggs on top of the toast with the cut melon on the side.

Skillet Eggs with Peppers and Herbs

SERVES 2

A Sunday brunch favorite, basted eggs (cooked in a covered pan) are cooked slightly more than sunny side up, with yolks that are set but not dried out. Serve with whole grain toast for a nutritious breakfast for two! Choosing omega-3-fortified eggs helps provide fatty acids that are essential for your baby's developing nervous system.

Olive oil spray
1 yellow bell pepper, stemmed, seeded, and diced
4 omega-3 eggs
2 tablespoons chopped fresh basil or parsley

Coat a large nonstick skillet with olive oil spray and cook the peppers over medium heat until soft. Make 4 wells in the peppers with a plastic spatula and crack an egg into each well. Cook until the whites are almost completely set, then cover the skillet and turn the heat down to low. Leave for 3 minutes, then check for doneness by poking one of the yolks. Cook 1 to 2 minutes longer if necessary. When done to your liking, sprinkle with the herbs and divide between two plates.

Week 11

(Gestational Week 13)

All of baby's essential organs and organ systems have formed.

What's Happening?

Your baby's head is now about half the size of its body, but not to worry—things will become more proportional. This week, the baby's small intestine is coiling around its umbilical cord outside its body (it will be brought inside later on). Also, your baby now looks more like a baby rather than an alien-like little being; it has visible hands and feet as well as teeny tiny fingers and toes. Your baby's facial features are developing as well, and the ears are nearly in their final place (they've been shifting up from the neck to the normal ear position). If you're expecting a girl, this is also a very important week, as her ovaries are now growing at full speed.

Food of the Week: Quinoa

Quinoa is a seed from South America that has surged in popularity in recent years due to its superior nutrition profile and great flavor. You may have heard quinoa referred to as a superfood. Living up to that name, quinoa is highly beneficial both now and later on in your pregnancy because it is simply packed with the nutrients you need. A cup of cooked quinoa has 40 g of carbohydrate, 5 g of fiber, and nearly 3 mg of iron, and is high in magnesium, phosphorus, potassium, and zinc; it also contains some folate and mono- as well as polyunsaturated fatty acids. You can eat quinoa as a main dish or as a side, as in this recipe. As with most foods, when it comes to staving off nausea, try eating quinoa cold if its smell is too overwhelming when hot. In addition to the recipe below, check out Rotisserie Chicken with Apricot Quinoa over Spinach (89).

Golden Quinoa with Raisins and Apricots

SERVES 2

Quinoa is as easy to cook as white rice, but has more flavor and higher amounts of iron, protein, fiber, and B vitamins. Try this dish served hot or cold—it is delicious both ways. Double or triple the recipe for a potluck, and everyone will want the recipe.

½ cup uncooked quinoa
1 cup water
6 dried apricots, chopped
2 tablespoons golden or dark raisins, not packed
⅓ teaspoon turmeric
¼ teaspoon salt
⅛ teaspoon cinnamon
Cayenne pepper to taste (optional)

Rinse the quinoa and combine it with the water in a saucepan. Bring to a boil over medium heat, then reduce to low, cover, and simmer for 15 minutes. Turn off the heat.

Stir the apricots, raisins, turmeric, salt, and cinnamon into the quinoa and let the mixture sit, covered, for 3 minutes. Taste and add cayenne if desired.

DO YOU REALLY NEED TO RINSE YOUR QUINOA?

There is a kitchen gadget for everything, but do you really need a quinoa strainer? Quinoa has a natural bitter coating of saponins, which give it a slight soaplike taste. Most people can't detect the soapy taste, but some are sensitive to it. Most commercially available quinoa comes prerinsed, but it doesn't hurt to give it a quick rinse anyway—an ordinary mesh kitchen strainer is all you need for this.

Week 12

(Gestational Week 14)

This is the last week of the first trimester. Your baby is now the size of a peach.

What's Happening?

Week 12 marks the end of the first trimester—you're now one-third of the way closer to meeting your baby! Most of your baby's organs are now working on their own, even as they continue to grow and develop at a fast pace. The intestines that were outside of its little body just last week are now neatly in place, tucked inside the abdomen. In addition, your baby is now producing certain hormones on its own, such as the pituitary hormone from the pituitary gland.

Food of the Week: Cod

Rich in protein, phosphorus, potassium, zinc, and vitamins B6, B12, and D, cod is an excellent lunch or dinner choice for this week. Your baby's growth is about to take off, big time, as you're entering the second trimester, and a lot of extra protein is needed to support it.

Cod with Roasted Red Pepper Sauce

SERVES 2

Cod is a white-fleshed, very mild-tasting fish. It is a rich source of protein and is low in mercury, making it a great pick for expectant moms. Use any leftover red pepper sauce as a dip for raw vegetables, or spread it on sandwiches instead of mayonnaise.

½ cup roasted red peppers, chopped
1 garlic clove
2 tablespoons low-fat mayonnaise
Salt and freshly ground black pepper
Cooking oil spray
2 cod fillets (¾ pound total)

Place the peppers, garlic, and mayo in a blender and puree until smooth. Season to taste with salt and pepper.

Spray a large skillet with cooking spray and place over medium-high heat. When hot, add the cod and season with salt and pepper. Cook until the bottom side is golden, 4 to 5 minutes, then reduce the heat to medium and flip the fillets. Cook until opaque throughout, 5 to 10 more minutes depending on the thickness of the fish. Serve with the red pepper sauce on the side.

Planning Out Your Meals

One of the best ways to ensure that you are eating well is to plan out a menu. Thinking ahead regarding what you plan to eat not only can save you time (and money) but also helps keep you on track with eating healthy foods and avoiding convenience foods (think vending-machine lunch at work). I offer a sample menu on the next page using the recipes in this chapter to give you a sense of how easy it is to get all of the essential nutrients that you and your baby need in this trimester by making a few quick and easy meals.

Keep this in mind: you don't need to stress about making sure you get enough of each and every nutrient *each day*; the key is to meet the recommended intakes of all nutrients over the course of two or three days. It is perfectly fine if your intake is a bit short or over the recommended amount, as long as the average is close to what is recommended. And know that exceeding the recommendations by consuming food sources alone is extremely unlikely to cause harm to you or your baby (seriously, it's just about impossible—the

One-Day Sample Menu for the First Trimester

Breakfast	Egg, Toast, and Melon plate (page 68) 1 cup orange juice (fortified with vitamin D and calcium)
Snack	8 ounces plain low-fat yogurt
Lunch	3 ounces cooked wild coho salmon ½ cup boiled spinach (no salt) 1 teaspoon extra-virgin olive oil
Snack	Banana and Almond Butter Wrap (page 63)
Dinner	Easy Seasoned Lentils (page 55) 1 cup raw kale 1 teaspoon extra-virgin olive oil
Snack	1 glass skim milk 2 ounces graham crackers (with honey)

Nutrient	Amount Needed Per Day	Provided by Menu
Carbohydrate	175 g	247 g
Protein	1.1 g per kg body weight	105 g
Fat	20% to 35% of total daily calories	73 g
Vitamin A	770 mcg RAE/2,565 IU	1,688 RAE
Vitamin B6	1.9 mg	2.76 mg
Vitamin B12	2.6 mcg	7.86 mcg
Vitamin C	85 mg	267 mg
Vitamin D	600 IU (15 mcg)	688 IU
Vitamin K	90 mcg	976 mcg
Calcium	1,000 mg	1,767 mg
Choline	450 mg	612 mg
EPA and DHA	350 mg EPA, 300 mg DHA	345 mg EPA, 597 mg DHA
Fiber	28 g	41 g
Folate/folic acid	600 DFE	930 DFE
Iron	27 mg	20.5 mg
Magnesium	350 to 360 mg	569 mg
Phosphorus	700 mg	2,214 mg
Potassium	4.7 g	5.2 g
Zinc	11 mg	12.4 mg

TOTAL ENERGY: 1,925 calories

rare exceptions are excess vitamin A in the form or retinol from animal sources such as liver). *Not* meeting the recommendations, on the other hand, can be more detrimental, so try your best to get what's needed, and if you're falling short, consider adding a supplement to fill in the nutritional gaps.

*　*　*

Can you believe you are already one-third of the way through your pregnancy? With the help of this chapter, your baby is off to a great start and growing strong because of the good food you are eating. In the next chapter, we will discuss which foods you need during the second trimester (otherwise known as the "honeymoon of pregnancy").

CHAPTER 5

The Second Trimester

Welcome to the middle of your pregnancy! Sometimes referred to as the "honeymoon of pregnancy," the second trimester is indeed an exciting time as well as a more relaxing one. Your baby will be growing very quickly in the next three months, and your belly will get oh-so-much-bigger than it is right now. However, despite the rapid baby and belly growth, you may feel close to ecstatic, as the hormone fluctuations, morning sickness, and food aversions that may have plagued you in the first trimester now remain at bay, allowing you to enjoy yourself more and truly bond with your baby. In addition, because all of your baby's organs have already formed, the developmental risks are significantly diminished compared to what they were in the first trimester (yet they still remain, so excellent nutrition is still key). Finally, after the 20th week, your baby will enter what is called the perinatal period, which will last until 7 days after birth.

Optimal Nutrition for the Honeymoon Period

Women often say the second trimester is the easiest of the three. The nausea and vomiting, food aversions, mood fluctuations, lack of energy, and all of the other not-so-great aspects of pregnancy that you may have gone through in the first three months have come to an end (or are fading and will end soon). At this point, you have also had some time to adapt to the changes your body has been going through, and your belly will now start expanding at a much faster pace. Your hormones will likely give you a sense of happiness and energy and make you feel more like yourself compared to the first three months. You're also most likely to experience the "pregnancy glow" during the second trimester, making it a perfect time to start planning the baby's room, celebrate with a baby shower, make arrangements at work for maternity leave, take a vacation (who wouldn't love a babymoon?), and—most important— really focus on superb nutrition.

With the morning sickness gone and your spirits higher, you may feel ready to enjoy more foods such as red meat, an increased variety of vegetables, and flavorful herbs and spices. The second trimester is a period of rapid growth during which your baby will get noticeably larger, so maintaining a balanced diet to support this growth is essential. The key vitamins, minerals, and nutrients that were highlighted for the first trimester remain important; in addition to these, optimal intake of protein, iron, calcium, and fiber are crucial in the second trimester.

The recipes included in this chapter will add more flavors back in, while keeping the focus on whole, nutrient-dense foods. Because of your increased needs for some new nutrients and minerals this trimester, the recipes will include a variety of iron- and protein-rich meats, as well as calcium- and fiber-rich foods, to help you and your growing baby stay well nourished. To further help you through your second trimester, you'll find filling soup recipes as well as ideas for how to make your own turkey and roast beef for sandwiches— deli meats are typically not recommended for expectant moms, due to the risk of listeriosis.

It's Time to Ramp Up (a Little) on Calories

Although you did not need additional calories to support your developing baby in the first trimester, you do need some extra energy now, as your baby's growth is about to really take off. However, as I mentioned earlier, you don't need to eat for two (contrary to that old saying). Throughout this trimester you need roughly 340 calories a day in addition to your normal daily calorie intake. These extra calories will help provide the extra nutrients that your growing baby and body need, as your breasts, uterus, placenta, and blood and amniotic fluid volume will all be increasing significantly during the next three months.

What does 340 calories look like? It really isn't a whole lot. To give you an idea of what is equivalent to 340 calories, here are a few examples:

3 medium/large bananas

4 ounces of mozzarella cheese (whole milk)

2 Luna bars

3 large apples

1½ wheat bagels (medium)

1½ avocados (medium)

1 peanut butter and jelly sandwich (2 slices of whole wheat bread, 1½ tablespoons of peanut butter, and 1 tablespoon of jelly)

About 2 ounces of raw cashew nuts

6.5 ounces of cooked Atlantic salmon

Your Second Trimester Week by Week

In the sections that follow, I discuss some of the key nutrients to focus on in the next three months and provide some delicious recipes for you and your growing baby. I also describe the developmental processes happening week by week so you know exactly what's happening in your belly.

Week 13

(Gestational Week 15)

Baby's growth takes off.

What's Happening?

Rapid growth is occurring now. Your baby's bones and more muscle tissue are developing, and the bones are becoming harder (a process called ossification). Interestingly, your baby is born with about 300 bones, which grow and fuse to eventually form the 206 bones of an adult. In addition, your baby is now growing some peach-fuzz-like body hair called lanugo, which will help it stay warm and cozy.

Food of the Week: Black Beans

Constipation may be setting in now, as hormones are relaxing your bowel's action. You should focus on consuming adequate amounts of fruits and veggies, as they contain loads of fiber (and don't forget liquids, especially water). Black beans are one of the best sources of fiber—1 cup of cooked beans contains about 15 g. In addition, it has nearly 41 g of healthy carbs, 15 g of protein, 3.6 mg of non-heme iron, 610 mg of potassium, 256 mcg of folate, and many other vitamins and minerals in moderate amounts. A healthy burrito made with black beans, black bean soup, or black beans as a side dish each will provide you with a large portion of your daily fiber needs.

Pork, Chard, and Black Bean Soup with Cumin

SERVES 4

If you don't have ancho chile powder, substitute smoked paprika. Longer simmering will make the pork more tender, so if you have time, let it cook for 60 minutes. Because this soup is low in fat, it doesn't sit heavily in your belly, but if you need to stay full for hours, pair it with some cheese and crackers.

6 cups low-sodium beef or chicken broth
4 white mushrooms, sliced
1 bunch Swiss chard (stems and leaves), chopped
½ yellow onion, chopped
1 (15-ounce) can no-salt-added black beans, drained and rinsed
1 (6-ounce) can no-salt-added tomato paste
1 pound pork tenderloin, cubed
1 tablespoon ground cumin
1 teaspoon ancho chile powder
½ teaspoon garlic powder
¼ teaspoon freshly ground black pepper

Combine all the ingredients in a large soup pot and bring to a boil. Reduce the heat to low and simmer for 30 minutes. Serve hot.

Week 14

(Gestational Week 16)

Listen closely: now you can hear your baby's heartbeat.

What's Happening?

If you have a check-up scheduled this week, you may hear your baby's heart-beat for the first time at your doctor's office. Make sure your partner comes along with you—this can be one of the most special moments during your pregnancy. In addition, if you're curious to find out whether you're expecting a boy or a girl, your doctor may be able to tell you the news this week (if you didn't find out during the first trimester), as your baby's genitals and reproductive organs are now fully formed. You may also feel increased movement in your belly since the baby can now move its arms and legs, suck its tiny thumb, and stretch, and it has a functioning nervous system. At week 14, your baby is around 8.5 centimeters long from crown to rump.

Food of the Week: Beef

Your iron needs are especially increased during this time, and beef is one of the best sources of iron, as it contains heme iron, which your body can absorb significantly better than iron from nonanimal sources. I encourage you to consume most, if not all, of your iron from food sources (fortified foods also count!) during the first and second trimesters (as research shows no benefit of supplementation if you are *not* iron-deficient), and choosing such high-iron sources as beef can significantly help you meet your iron needs by diet alone. A 4-ounce serving of beef brisket can provide about 3 mg of iron and 30 g of protein, as well as significant amounts of phosphorus, potassium, zinc, niacin, and vitamin B12. When buying and cooking beef at home or ordering at a restaurant, go for the leaner cuts instead of those with more fat—although high in numerous beneficial vitamins and nutrients, fatty cuts are also high in cholesterol and provide excess calories. In addition to the recipes below, check out Slow Cooker BBQ-Salsa Chicken (page 120).

Beef and Mushroom Soup with Barley

SERVES 2 TO 3 AS AN ENTRÉE, 4 TO 6 AS A SIDE

This soup pairs iron-rich beef with high-fiber barley in a comforting, belly-filling meal. We recommend serving it alongside a green salad for a perfect lunch. It's freezer friendly too, in case you want to make it ahead of time, or double the amount and freeze two-serving portions to be thawed and heated in the future.

1½ teaspoons extra-virgin olive oil
1½ teaspoons butter
8 ounces mixed mushrooms, sliced
½ yellow onion, chopped
1 pound lean beef cubes (can use leftover steak or roast beef)
4 cups beef broth
1 cup water
½ teaspoon ground dried rosemary
½ teaspoon garlic powder
¼ cup uncooked barley

In a large soup pot, heat the olive oil and butter over medium-low heat for 2 minutes. Add the mushrooms and onion and cook, stirring occasionally, for 10 minutes or until soft and fragrant. Add the beef, broth, water, rosemary, garlic, and barley and bring the soup to a boil. Reduce the heat to low and simmer for 60 minutes. Serve hot.

Best Beef Burgers

SERVES 4

Iron-rich beef helps prevent anemia during pregnancy and is a source of high-quality protein and vitamin B12. Serve these with whole grain buns and, if you like, top them with cheese for an extra calcium boost.

1 pound extra-lean ground beef
½ cup finely diced onion
½ teaspoon salt
¼ teaspoon freshly ground black pepper
½ teaspoon Worcestershire sauce
2 teaspoons Dijon mustard
1 egg white

Combine all of the ingredients in a bowl and mix well. Form the mixture into 4 burgers. Grill until the internal temperature reaches 165°F.

Lean Roast Beef "Deli Meat"

SERVES 6 TO 8 (ABOUT 4 OUNCES EACH)

If you are used to buying roast beef for sandwiches from the deli counter, the recommendation to avoid deli meats can come as a disappointment. But don't worry; making your own roast beef is so easy (and much cheaper than buying it at the deli counter) that you might keep making your own from now on!

1 teaspoon ground dried rosemary
1 teaspoon garlic powder
1 teaspoon onion powder
¾ teaspoon salt
½ teaspoon freshly ground black pepper
1 tablespoon prepared mustard (yellow or Dijon)
1 tablespoon extra-virgin olive oil
1½ to 2 pounds lean beef round roast

Preheat the oven to 375°F.

Combine the rosemary, garlic, onion, salt, and pepper in a small bowl. Add the mustard and olive oil and stir to make a paste. Rub the mixture over all sides of the beef roast.

Insert a meat thermometer into the center of the thickest part of the roast and place the roast in a roasting pan. Bake until the internal temperature of the meat reaches 130°F, about 60 minutes.

Remove from the oven, cover with foil, and allow to rest for at least 10 minutes. Slice and serve hot, or refrigerate for up to 5 days and use in sandwiches.

Week 15

(Gestational Week 17)

Here comes the baby fat.

What's Happening?

This week, your baby's fat stores begin to form, which will help regulate metabolism and heat production. When the baby is born it will experience its greatest temperature shock, being immediately exposed to the relatively cool surroundings outside of the womb. Adipose—or fat—tissue, especially brown adipose tissue, will help your baby survive this change by producing sufficient heat to maintain body temperature in a new environment and keep its tiny body warm. Adipose tissue will continue to form until week 18.

Food of the Week: Chicken

A great source of protein, iron, and B vitamins, chicken is an excellent choice in the second trimester. A 4-ounce roasted chicken breast (no skin) has 35 g of protein and 1.2 mg of iron and is also high in phosphorus, potassium, zinc, and niacin. You can enjoy it both as a main dish as well as part of a soup or salad. Just remember to always choose lean chicken and remove the skin before eating, as the skin is high in both calories and cholesterol. In addition to the recipes below, check out Rotisserie Chicken with Apricot Quinoa over Spinach (page 89), Roasted or Raw Beet Salad (page 60), and the week 34 chicken recipes beginning on page 120.

Lemony Grilled Chicken Kabobs

SERVES 6

This recipe is one your whole family will love. It's simple and easy, but plan ahead so the chicken has time to soak and absorb the flavors in the marinade.

Juice from 1 lemon
2 tablespoons extra-virgin olive oil
½ tablespoon red wine vinegar
1½ teaspoons dried oregano
½ teaspoon salt
⅛ teaspoon freshly ground black pepper
1½ pounds skinless boneless chicken breast, cubed

Mix the lemon juice, olive oil, vinegar, oregano, salt, and pepper in a plastic resealable bag. Add the chicken to the bag and marinate for at least 2 hours, preferably overnight.

Preheat a grill. Thread the chicken cubes onto metal or bamboo skewers and grill to an internal temperature of 165°F.

Savory Roasted Chicken Breasts
with Whole Grain Mustard

SERVES 6

Bone-in chicken breasts are less expensive than skinless boneless breasts, and cooking them in the oven is a breeze. Just put them in, then relax for half an hour or so until they are done. We recommend making plenty of extra, as the leftover meat can be sliced thin and used for sandwiches. If you prefer turkey, bone-in turkey breast also works with this recipe; it will just take longer to cook because of the larger size.

2 pounds bone-in skinless chicken or turkey breast
Olive oil cooking spray
¾ teaspoon salt
½ teaspoon freshly ground black pepper
1½ teaspoons onion powder
1½ teaspoons garlic powder
1½ teaspoons paprika (regular, not hot)
Whole grain mustard

Preheat the oven to 400°F. Line a baking sheet with foil and arrange the chicken on top.

Lightly spray the chicken with olive oil spray, and sprinkle with the salt, pepper, onion powder, garlic powder, and paprika.

Bake small chicken breasts for 30 minutes, large ones for 40 minutes, or until the temperature in the thickest part reaches 165°F. Allow to rest for 5 minutes before slicing and serving with whole grain mustard.

Chicken Thighs with Spicy Peanut Sauce

SERVES 4

Try this flavorful, Thai-inspired chicken with rice or quinoa and steamed broccoli. If you have cilantro on hand, a little sprinkle on top adds an attractive and flavorful finish.

1 cup chicken broth
¼ cup natural peanut butter
1 tablespoon honey
2 teaspoons soy sauce

⅛ to ¼ teaspoon cayenne pepper (for milder heat, use ⅛ teaspoon;
  you can always add more)
8 boneless, skinless chicken thighs (about 1½ pounds total)
Salt and freshly ground black pepper

In a small saucepan, combine the broth, peanut butter, honey, soy sauce, and cayenne. Stir and bring to a boil over medium-high heat, then reduce the heat to medium-low and simmer for 10 minutes. Keep the sauce hot until serving time.

Lightly season the chicken thighs with salt and pepper. Heat a large skillet over medium-high heat and add 4 chicken thighs in a single layer. Cook for 5 to 6 minutes on each side, until both sides are a rich golden brown. Transfer to a clean plate and cook the remaining 4 pieces of chicken in the same manner.

Place 2 chicken thighs per person on serving plates and pour the sauce over the chicken.

Week 16

(Gestational Week 18)

Your baby is now approximately 5 inches long and weighs 5 ounces.

What's Happening?

Your baby continues to grow quickly and is now capable of a variety of expressions, including smiling, frowning, yawning, stretching, and even hiccupping. Its taste buds are starting to develop, and it can now tell sweet and bitter flavors apart when swallowing tiny bits of amniotic fluid. In addition, your baby's eyes are now developed enough for it to react to light—if your abdomen is exposed to a bright light, you may feel your baby react and move to protect its eyes! However, its movements at this small size may still be too faint for you to feel for another couple of weeks. Your baby may also begin to hear this week, as its ears have (or have nearly) reached their final position on the sides of its head.

Food of the Week: Almonds

Rich in healthy fats and a variety of vitamins and minerals, almonds are an excellent choice this week. Two ounces can provide you with 2.1 mg of iron (non-heme), 12 g of protein, 28 g of healthy fats including mono- and poly-unsaturated fatty acids, 7 g of fiber, and 14.5 mg of vitamin E, as well as moderate quantities of calcium, magnesium, phosphorus, potassium, zinc, niacin, and riboflavin.

You may be experiencing sudden bursts of hunger or cravings, so it is a good idea to always carry some snacks in your purse—and raw, unsalted almonds are a great choice. However, remember that just like all nuts, almonds are also high in calories; a 2-ounce portion contains nearly 340 calories, the full allowance of the recommended extra daily calories for the second trimester. Here are some other ways you can slip some almonds into your daily routine: add a few crushed or slivered almonds to a salad instead of croutons, use them as a topping on your yogurt, or add some sliced almonds to a sautéed vegetable dish. In addition to the recipe below, check out Marinated Wasabi Steak with Brown Rice Pilaf (page 114).

No-Bake Honey Almond Cereal Bars

SERVES 9

These crispy whole grain cereal bars have much less sugar than store-bought granola bars, and with just a few ingredients, they are a snap to make. You can use peanut butter or sunflower seed butter for a different flavor or if you have nut allergies in your household. Try them frozen; they are extra-satisfying to gnaw on straight from the freezer.

¼ cup honey
¼ cup almond butter
¼ cup dark chocolate chips
3 cups Multigrain or Original Cheerios (or similar whole grain, low-sugar cereal)

Line a 9 by 9-inch baking pan with parchment paper.

In a small saucepan over medium-low heat, combine the honey, almond butter, and chocolate chips. Stir and cook until the chocolate is melted and the mixture is smooth. Turn off the heat.

Put the Cheerios into a large mixing bowl and pour in the honey mixture, stirring to coat the cereal. Press into the prepared pan and refrigerate for 2 hours or until firm. Cut into 9 squares. Keep prepared bars wrapped in plastic or freeze for longer-term storage.

DOES ALMOND MILK HAVE THE SAME BENEFITS AS WHOLE ALMONDS?

The answer is both yes and no. Half a cup (46 g) of whole almonds contains more energy, protein, fat, fiber, iron, magnesium, phosphorus, potassium, and vitamin D, as well as mono- and polyunsaturated fatty acids compared to an 8-ounce glass of almond milk. However, the latter has its own benefits—it is much higher in calcium than whole almonds (a single glass provides nearly half of your daily calcium requirement), zinc, and vitamins A, B12, and D (the vitamins are added in the process of making the milk)—in addition to containing all the nutrients that whole almonds do, albeit in smaller amounts. Almond milk also contains added vitamin E; 1 cup contains nearly half of your daily recommendation, making it an excellent source of antioxidants. Bottom line: both almonds and almond milk are great choices, even though they differ in their nutrient composition and therefore provide slightly different nutritional benefits. However, be aware that some varieties of almond milk may be high in added sugars. Always check the label and choose those with the lowest amount. In addition, keep in mind that almond milk, just like any other tree nut products, is off-limits if you have tree nut allergies.

Week 17

(Gestational Week 19)

Baby's skin is developing.

What's Happening?

Your baby's skin is developing, and if you were able to see it, it would appear transparent and red, as you could see right through it, revealing the blood vessels beneath the surface. To protect this very delicate skin from the chapping that would result from soaking in the amniotic fluid, a creamy protective coating called *vernix caseosa* begins to develop, which will continue to cover your baby's entire body until birth. In addition, if you're expecting a girl, her uterus is forming this week.

Food of the Week: Chocolate

Your body is hard at work supporting your baby's rapid growth, and combined with the cravings that you may be experiencing now—mama, you need a break! While chocolate is generally a dessert item (often combined with full-fat dairy, butter, and sugar) and should be consumed in moderation, dark chocolate offers several health benefits and contains important nutrients, such as iron, magnesium, phosphorus, potassium, zinc, niacin, and monounsaturated fatty acids. Recent research shows that a modest intake of high-cacao chocolate (30 g of at least 70-percent cacao chocolate) can help reduce blood pressure and improve insulin sensitivity during pregnancy without affecting weight gain. However, remember that even though it is beneficial, chocolate is high in calories and fat and contains caffeine, so indulge in moderation. Try to keep your intake at or under 1 ounce of high-quality dark chocolate per day, and aim for dark chocolate with 70- to 85-percent cacao solids. The recipes for Chocolate Oat Bran with Peanut Butter (below) and Frozen Banana–Peanut Butter–Chocolate Bites (page 88) may inspire other creative and delicious ways to add chocolate to your diet. In addition to the recipes below, check out No-Bake Honey Almond Cereal Bars (page 85).

Chocolate Oat Bran with Peanut Butter

SERVES 2

Chocolate and peanut butter are two of the foods that expectant mothers most commonly crave. Here you can satisfy your hankerings for both with a big filling bowl of sweet, chocolatey hot cereal. Your sweet tooth will never know you are also getting protein, B vitamins, calcium, and fiber. We won't tell.

1 cup oat bran
Pinch of salt
4 tablespoons unsweetened cocoa powder
Sugar or other sweetener to taste
4 cups skim, 1%, or almond milk
4 tablespoons peanut butter

Combine the oat bran, salt, cocoa, sugar, and milk in a small saucepan over medium-high heat. Bring it to a boil, stirring, then reduce the heat to low and simmer for 4 minutes. To serve, pour the cereal into 2 bowls and top with the peanut butter.

Frozen Banana-Chocolate-Peanut Butter Bites

SERVES 2

Depending on personal preference, you may find that you like these best after more or less time in the freezer. Following these directions, they will be fully frozen, but some people prefer them partially frozen or not frozen at all. For those with nut allergies, omit the peanut butter and sprinkle the melted chocolate with crisp rice cereal for a crunchy treat.

1 banana, sliced into about 12 slices
1 tablespoon peanut butter
1 ounce chocolate chips

Place the banana slices on a plate lined with wax paper. Spread each slice with a small amount of peanut butter. Put the plate in the freezer to chill.

Microwave the chocolate chips in 30-second intervals, stirring between, until melted and smooth. Smear a little melted chocolate on top of each banana slice. Freeze for at least 2 hours and up to 24 hours.

Week 18

(Gestational Week 20)

Welcome to the midpoint of your pregnancy.

What's Happening?

Your baby has nearly doubled in size in the past two weeks and now weighs about 9 ounces. Its ears are fully developed, and it can hear—and react to—the sounds it is exposed to, in both your body and the wider environment. Your voice, heartbeat, and digestive sounds, your conversations with others, music, and other noises—your baby is listening to all of it and may even move or kick in response! These first movements are called quickening; you may or may not have felt them a week or even a few weeks ago; if not, it is likely that this week you will experience them for the first time.

Food of the Week: Dried Fruits

Great sources of non-heme iron, dried fruits such as apricots, raisins, dates, and others can provide the nutrients and fiber that your body needs at this time.

A cup of muesli with dried fruits and nuts can supply about 40 percent of your iron needs and also contains more than 400 mg of potassium, more than 60 g of carbohydrates, 6 g of fiber, vitamin A, and protein. You can make your own dried fruit mix at home and carry a small container around with you to snack on. As with chocolate, it's important to remember to consume dried fruits in moderation; they generally contain high amounts of sugar and calories. Also, when looking at ingredient labels, make sure that they're unsweetened and unsalted. In addition to the recipe below, check out Stuffed Portobello Caps with Wild Rice, Cherries, and Pecans (page 114).

Rotisserie Chicken with Apricot Quinoa over Spinach

SERVES 4

A quick side dish paired with a rotisserie chicken makes for an easy meal, plus there's only one pot to wash when you're done. The sweetness of apricots partners beautifully with curry powder in the quinoa, and wilting spinach in the microwave is a speedy shortcut for upping the folate in this weeknight-friendly meal.

2 cups water
1 cup quinoa
4 dried apricots, finely chopped
2 teaspoons curry powder
½ teaspoon salt
1 store-bought rotisserie chicken, skinned (skin discarded)
1 (5-ounce) bag baby spinach

In a saucepan, bring the water to a boil over high heat. Add the quinoa, apricots, curry powder, and salt. Cover and reduce the heat to low. Simmer for 15 minutes, then turn off the heat and allow the quinoa to steam for 5 more minutes.

While the quinoa cooks, put 4 ounces of cooked meat onto each of 4 plates. (Refrigerate the leftover chicken for another meal.) You can keep the plates warm in the oven set to the lowest temperature, if needed.

When the quinoa is ready, place a big handful of the spinach on each plate and microwave for 45 seconds to wilt. Place the quinoa on top of the spinach and serve.

A balanced mix of dried fruits, such as in a breakfast muesli, will provide a generous amount of non-heme iron, usually around 40 percent of your recommended daily allowance. However, different types of dried fruits eaten separately do differ in their iron content. Half a cup of dried Zante currants has 2.35 mg of iron, apricots 1.73 mg, raisins 1.55 mg, figs 1.51 mg, prunes 0.81 mg, and dates 0.75 mg. However, keep in mind that some dried fruits can be very high in sugar, so what you "win" in gaining more iron, you'll "lose" in getting too much sugar. Dried fruits with particularly high sugar content include cranberries (which generally have added sweetener; they are otherwise too sour), pineapple, and banana chips. In addition to added sugar, banana chips are frequently deep-fried; however, there are unsweetened and nonfried versions, so keep your eyes out for some healthy dried banana chips (freeze-dried ones are light and crunchy) next time you're in the grocery store if you enjoy your bananas dried—just don't forget to eat some fresh ones, too!

Week 19

(Gestational Week 21)

Baby's organs continue to mature this week.

What's Happening?

Your baby continues to grow in size and weight, and even though the growth rate is slowing down a bit, its organ systems are diligently maturing and becoming more sophisticated every day. This week, buds for your baby's permanent teeth are forming, and the digestive system continues to prepare for processing food taken in by mouth and eliminating waste after birth.

Food of the Week: Cheese

To supply the calcium needed for the healthy bone and tooth development that is now taking place, it is very important to ensure that you are getting enough calcium in your diet. Most cheeses are great sources, and Swiss is one of the best. Two ounces contain almost half your daily calcium needs (438 mg), as well as lots of protein (14 g), phosphorus, zinc, potassium, and vitamins A and B12. However, cheese can also be high in sodium (the same 2 ounces of regular Swiss has almost 780 mg, a third of your daily limit of salt intake), so keep your intake moderate, and if possible, choose lower-sodium cheeses. In addition, remember to consume only pasteurized (and in most cases, hard) cheeses, due to the potential risks of foodborne illnesses. You don't have to avoid or be scared of cheese in general. As long as it's made from pasteurized milk (most store-bought cheese or cheese served in restaurants is pasteurized; see Appendix A for more on pasteurized dairy products), foodborne risks associated with cheese are the same as with most other foods. In addition to the recipes below, check out Turkey-Apple Burgers with Cheddar (page 99); Anchovy, Parsley, and Parmesan Cheese Quiche (page 112); and Roasted or Raw Beet Salad (page 60).

Two-Pepper Turkey and Havarti Sandwich with Radish Salad

SERVES 2

Once you've made your own lunch meat, sandwiches are back on the menu! This tasty combination pairs sweet peppers, hot peppers, and creamy Havarti for a perfect lunch. It's not only delicious, but also a well-rounded meal with protein, calcium, fiber, and complex carbohydrates.

4 slices whole wheat bread
8 ounces roasted sliced turkey breast (homemade)
2 large roasted red peppers (jarred)
4 tablespoons banana pepper rings (jarred)
2 slices Havarti cheese
2 cups sliced radishes
½ cup plain Greek yogurt
½ teaspoon dried dill
Salt and freshly ground black pepper

Toast the bread slices and make 2 sandwiches by layering the turkey, roasted red peppers, banana pepper rings, and Havarti.

In a bowl, add the radishes with the yogurt and dill and stir to combine. Add salt and pepper to taste. Serve alongside the sandwich.

Spaghetti Squash with Basil, Cheese, and Sun-Dried Tomatoes

SERVES 4

Spaghetti squash shines when served with classic Italian flavors. Cooking the squash in the microwave before mixing with the other ingredients saves time.

1 spaghetti squash
½ cup shredded fresh basil
½ cup coarsely chopped sun-dried tomatoes
1 teaspoon salt
1 teaspoon garlic powder
½ teaspoon freshly ground black pepper
1 ounce mozzarella cheese, grated
1 ounce Parmesan cheese, grated

Preheat the oven to 400°F. Cut the squash in half and scrape out the seeds.

Place the squash halves, cut-side down, on a plate and microwave for 5 minutes. (Allow the squash to cool inside the microwave for a few minutes before handling.)

While the squash cools, combine the basil, sun-dried tomatoes, salt, garlic powder, and pepper in a large mixing bowl. Scrape the squash strands into the mixing bowl and toss to combine. Add the mozzarella and fold gently into the squash. Spread the squash mixture into a 9 by 13-inch baking dish and sprinkle with the Parmesan cheese. Bake for 10 minutes, then serve warm.

Week 20

(Gestational Week 22)

Move, kick, stretch: there are a lot of intrauterine acrobatics going on this week.

What's Happening?

Your baby's muscles are growing and becoming stronger every day, and your baby is now moving, kicking, stretching, and generally responding to sounds, flavors, light, and touch. It can now feel and experience all these stimuli. In addition, your baby's entire little body is covered in fine, fur-like lanugo hair, which started to grow a few weeks ago (don't worry—if you carry your baby to term, it will usually be shed by the time it is born). In addition to providing some warmth, this hair helps your baby hold the vernix coating on its body to protect its delicate skin. Eyebrows are now growing as well. At 20 weeks, your baby's body is about 19 centimeters long.

Food of the Week: Pork

Even though pork is often stigmatized, leaner varieties of pork (although "leaner" is a relative term when talking about pork), such as pork tenderloin, actually contain many valuable vitamins and minerals. A 4-ounce roasted lean tenderloin contains 1.15 mg of heme iron and 30 g of protein, as well as phosphorus, potassium, zinc, thiamin, niacin, and vitamins B6 and B12. Choose healthy, low-fat pork cuts to make sure that the many vitamins and nutrients pork contains are not accompanied by too many calories and grams of fat. In addition to the recipe below, check out Roast Pork Tenderloin with Apples, Squash, and Golden Raisins (page 117) and Pork, Chard, and Black Bean Soup with Cumin (page 78).

Grilled Pork Tenderloin with Peach-Jalapeño Salsa

SERVES 2 TO 4

Pork tenderloin can be almost as lean as chicken breast, and it resists drying out better than pork loin chops. The peach-jalapeño salsa is also delicious spooned over grilled chicken or fish, so feel free to try it alongside other meats at your next barbecue.

1 large peach, finely chopped
¼ cup finely chopped sweet onion
1 jalapeño, seeded and finely chopped
Pinch of salt
2 teaspoons freshly squeezed lime juice
1 large (¾- to 1-pound) pork tenderloin, cut in half lengthwise
Salt and freshly ground black pepper

In a mixing bowl, combine the peach, onion, jalapeño, salt, and lime juice and stir until well blended. Refrigerate for at least 1 hour.

Preheat an indoor or outdoor grill. Season both sides of the pork lightly with salt and pepper and grill until the internal temperature reaches 160°F.

Slice the pork and serve with the salsa spooned over it.

Week 21

(Gestational Week 23)

You've hit 1 pound, baby!

What's Happening?

As you can most likely tell from your nice round belly, your baby has dramatically increased in size and now weighs about 1 pound. Its body is getting more and more proportional each day, with the head now appearing smaller compared to the rest of the body (whew!). Fingerprints (and footprints) have now formed, with patterns entirely unique to your baby. In addition, if you're expecting a girl, her ovaries are now formed and in place, along with all the eggs she will ever have during her lifetime. Finally, your baby has now entered the perinatal period, which will last from this point until it is born and is about 1 week old.

Food of the Week: Raspberries

High in fiber, vitamins C and K, and manganese, raw raspberries can not only help with constipation but also may provide some elasticity to your stretching skin due to their vitamin C content. A cup of fresh raspberries contains 8 g of fiber, 12 g of carbohydrates, 0.69 mg of iron, 26 mg of vitamin C, and has moderate amounts of vitamin K, folate, niacin, zinc, and potassium. You can indulge in raspberries either on their own or as part of a fruit smoothie with raspberries, blackberries, kiwis, mangos, blueberries, and bananas. And when fresh raspberries are out of season, look for frozen; they thaw quickly and easily.

If you're a smoothie fan, you may be acquainted with some delicious smoothie recipes already, but if you're not, this is the perfect time to become a smoothie expert! I recommend the Ninja or the NutriBullet blenders. Both are convenient, relatively inexpensive, easy to clean, and overall awesome blenders. You can make your own nutrient-packed smoothies that will provide you with loads of vitamins, minerals, and—very important—fiber, which is lost entirely when you drink juice (a good reason to choose smoothies over juices, at least most of the time). I've included two smoothie recipes here, but try out your own combos, too!

Raspberry Pear Smoothie

Pairing a tart berry with a sweet fruit makes for a balanced, delicious drink. Add whey protein if you want extra nourishment.

1 cup fresh or frozen raspberries
1 cup unsweetened almond milk or cow's milk
1 pear, core removed (peel if desired, or leave the peel for extra fiber)
6 ice cubes
1 scoop whey protein powder (optional)

Blend all ingredients until smooth.

Summer Fruit Smoothie

SERVES 1 TO 2

This nutritious fruit smoothie is a quick and easy way to get vitamin C, fiber, and potassium in a form you can drink anywhere, even if you're running out the door. Feel free to vary the types of fruit to suit your own taste.

¼ cup each raspberries, blackberries, apple, blueberries, kiwi, strawberries
8 ounces skim milk (or almond, soy, or hemp milk)
2 ounces low-fat yogurt

Blend all ingredients until smooth.

Week 22

(Gestational Week 24)

Baby's immune system is developing this week.

What's Happening?

Your baby's bone marrow is now actively producing the white blood cells that are part of the immune system and will help it fight infections. In addition, the lower airways of baby's lungs develop, even though they are not yet working in the same way as your lungs (they will start to immediately after birth).

The hair on your baby's head is now also growing, and baby has developed a regular sleeping and waking pattern—although not necessarily similar to your own (if only!). At 22 weeks, your baby is around 27 centimeters long—almost a foot.

Food of the Week: Broccoli

Broccoli is a great option either raw or cooked, and it can be eaten as part of a salad or as a side dish. If you are experiencing leg cramps now, broccoli may be especially helpful because its high potassium content can help alleviate this symptom. One cup of raw broccoli contains nearly 300 mg of potassium, 81 mg of vitamin C, 28 mcg of vitamin A, 92.5 mcg of vitamin K, as well as moderate amounts of fiber, folate, and iron. The following recipe is a real nutrient bomb.

Roasted Broccoli, Brussels Sprouts, and Carrot with Paprika

SERVES 2

Having steamed veggies every day can get boring. Roasting vegetables with olive oil bring them to a whole new level of deliciousness, caramelizing the natural sugars and giving them irresistible crispy golden spots.

1 broccoli crown (about 1 pound)
½ pound brussels sprouts
1 carrot
½ yellow onion
2 teaspoons extra-virgin olive oil
Paprika
Salt to taste

Preheat the oven to 350°F and line a baking sheet with foil.

Cut the broccoli into long thin pieces so that the stems are no thicker than a finger. Cut the brussels sprouts in half. Cut the carrot and onion into strips. Put all of the vegetables in a mixing bowl and add the oil. Toss to coat. Spread the vegetables in a single layer on the baking sheet and sprinkle lightly with paprika and salt. Bake for 45 minutes or until tender.

Week 23

(Gestational Week 25)

Your baby is about 1½ pounds and growing.

What's Happening?

Your baby's skin is undergoing more changes; still wrinkly-looking and covered in the creamy white coating of vernix, it is becoming more opaque. Your baby now weighs a little more than 1½ pounds and is continuing to grow and develop.

Food of the Week: Yogurt

Your baby's bones need plenty of calcium to support their growth. Yogurt, especially low-fat or fat-free, is an excellent choice both to supply needed calcium for your baby and to nourish your own body without adding excess calories. A 6-ounce cup of plain low-fat yogurt contains 311 mg of calcium, 9 g of protein, 12 g of carbs, and 400 mg of potassium and is also a good source of phosphorus, zinc, and vitamin B12. If you don't fancy plain yogurt, no worries: add some fresh fruit (either raw, or try pureeing your favorite ones) or a drizzle of honey. These add-ins will increase the flavor dramatically and make it a truly delicious snack! In addition to the recipe below, check out Two-Pepper Turkey and Havarti Sandwich with Radish Salad (page 91) and Summer Fruit Smoothie (page 95).

Sweet Stuffed Winter Squash with Coconut and Yogurt

SERVES 2

This sweet and satisfying meal idea helps you increase your intake of nutrient-dense foods like squash, yogurt, and nut butter. The harmony of decadent flavors is accompanied by vitamin A, calcium, protein, and healthy fat.

1 small carnival, delicata, or acorn squash
1 cup plain 2% fat Greek yogurt
Sweetener of choice (Splenda, stevia, honey, maple syrup, agave)
2 tablespoons natural peanut butter or almond butter
2 tablespoons milk or almond milk

2 tablespoons unsweetened shredded coconut
Pumpkin pie spice

Preheat the oven to 350°F and grease or oil a roasting dish.

Slice the squash in half and scoop out the seeds. Place both halves face down in the roasting dish and roast for 45 minutes to 1 hour (depending on size), until tender.

Mix the yogurt with sweetener to taste and fill the inside of the still-warm squash halves. Combine the nut butter and milk in a small bowl and microwave for 20 seconds. Stir, then drizzle over the filled squash halves. Sprinkle with coconut and pumpkin pie spice.

Week 24

(Gestational Week 26)

Let's dance: your baby is really starting to move!

What's Happening?

Because your baby's hearing is fully developed and its reflexes have been improving with each day, you may frequently feel it move in response to sounds, voices, and music. If you're dancing around the house listening to your favorite song, you're likely not alone—your little "partner" may be kicking and wiggling to the rhythm along with you! In addition, your baby has doubled in weight since week 21 and now weighs close to 2 pounds.

Food of the Week: Apples

Another great source of fiber and many vitamins, an apple (or two) a day will help keep constipation away. A large apple with skin has 5.4 g of fiber, 30 g of healthy carbs, 240 g of potassium, 7 mcg of vitamin A, 10.3 mg of vitamin C, and nearly 5 mcg of vitamin K. Remember to leave the skin on: that's where the majority of the fiber and vitamins reside. It's also a good idea to carry an apple with you in your bag. It's a healthy and nutrient-packed snack that will provide many of the vitamins and nutrients you need without adding too many calories (a large apple has just over 100 calories). In addition to the recipe below, check out Roast Pork Tenderloin with Apples, Squash, and Golden Raisins (page 117) and Summer Fruit Smoothie (page 95).

Turkey-Apple Burgers with Cheddar

SERVES 4

Tired of the same old burgers? Mix up these turkey burgers and love your burgers again. These lean turkey burgers have a flavor reminiscent of turkey-apple sausage. With cheddar melted on top, they are a real treat!

1 pound lean ground turkey (93% or 99% lean)
1 cup finely diced Fuji apple (1 medium)
½ cup minced yellow onion (½ medium)
1 teaspoon dried rubbed sage
1 teaspoon salt
¼ teaspoon garlic powder
¼ teaspoon freshly ground black pepper
⅛ teaspoon ground nutmeg
⅛ teaspoon ground allspice
1 egg
4 tablespoons grated cheddar cheese
4 whole wheat hamburger buns
Lettuce (optional)
Tomato slices (optional)

Put the turkey in a large mixing bowl and sprinkle the apple, onion, sage, salt, garlic powder, pepper, nutmeg, and allspice over the top. Add the egg and mix thoroughly. Divide and shape the mixture into 4 patties, about 1 inch thick.

Heat a large nonstick skillet over medium heat for 1 minute, then add the burgers. Depending on the size of your skillet, you may be able to cook only 2 at a time. Cook the burgers for 5 minutes, then turn them over and cover the skillet. Cook for 5 minutes more, then top each burger with 1 tablespoon of the cheese. Cover the skillet again for 1 minute to melt the cheese.

Serve the burgers in the buns with lettuce and tomato, if desired.

Week 25

(Gestational Week 27)

In the final week of the second trimester, your baby reaches another milestone: it is 1 foot long.

What's Happening?

This week is your baby's last in the second trimester. It is actively developing facial, cheek, and jaw muscles and may be exercising them by actively sucking a thumb, which is also considered a calming strategy (just as it will be outside the womb). In addition, your baby's lungs and brain continue to develop. Your baby has also tripled in length since the end of the first trimester; it is now a foot long and weighs about 2 pounds.

Food of the Week: Avocado

Rich in the "good" fats (mono- and polyunsaturated fatty acids) and numerous vitamins and minerals, avocado is a true nutritional powerhouse and an outstanding food choice at this time. One avocado (about 200 g) contains nearly 30 g of healthy fat, 17 g of carbs, 163 mcg of folate, 1.11 mg of iron, almost a quarter of your daily potassium needs (975 mcg), 20 mg of vitamin C, 14 mcg of vitamin A, more than 4 mg of vitamin E, 42 mcg of vitamin K, and moderate amounts of many other vitamins and minerals. Choose salads with avocado, add it to a sandwich, or enjoy guacamole with some tortilla chips. No matter what you choose, you will get a delicious, nutrient-packed meal or snack. In addition to the recipe below, check out Mom-Safe Sushi Bowl (page 107); Shrimp and Mango Kabobs (page 129); and Arugula Salad with Turkey, Avocado, and Dried Cranberries (page 65).

Shrimp, Avocado, and Cilantro Salad

SERVES 2 TO 3 AS AN ENTRÉE, 6 TO 8 AS AN APPETIZER

This salad will melt in your mouth. Serve it with mixed greens or cooked, chilled pasta for a refreshing summer meal, or in endive leaves for elegant appetizers that are deceptively easy and quick to prepare.

1 pound cooked shrimp (salad shrimp or any other size)
Juice from 1 lime
½ cup chopped cilantro
1 avocado, cubed
½ cup thinly sliced red onion
1 jalapeño, seeded and finely chopped (optional)

Combine all the ingredients in a large bowl and stir to mix well. Enjoy immediately or allow the salad to marinate in the refrigerator for up to 48 hours.

One-Day Sample Menu for the Second Trimester

Breakfast	Summer Fruit Smoothie (16 ounces; page 95) ¾ cup fortified breakfast cereal (such as Kellogg's All-Bran Complete Wheat Flakes)
Snack	Frozen Banana–Chocolate–Peanut Butter Bites (page 88)
Lunch	3 ounces Lean Roast Beef "Deli Meat" (page 81) 2½ cups Roasted Broccoli, Brussels Sprouts, and Carrot with Paprika (page 96) 1 tablespoon extra-virgin olive oil added to ½ cup black beans ½ cup light vanilla ice cream
Snack	1 whole grain granola bar (such as Kind Maple Pumpkin Seed Bar) ½ cup cottage cheese
Dinner	Shrimp, Avocado, and Cilantro Salad (page 100) 2 pieces whole wheat toast 1 cup orange juice (fortified with vitamin D and calcium)
Snack	1 ounce each of Swiss cheese cubes, whole raw almonds, and dried apricots

Nutrient	Amount Needed Per Day	Provided by Menu
Carbohydrate	175 g	270 g
Protein	1.1 g per kg body weight	127 g
Fat	20% to 35% of total daily calories	92 g
Vitamin A	770 mcg RAE/2,565 IU	1,196 mcg RAE
Vitamin B6	1.9 mg	4.58 mg
Vitamin B12	2.6 mcg	12.2 mcg
Vitamin C	85 mg	403 mg
Vitamin D	600 IU (15 mcg)	268 IU
Vitamin K	90 mcg	467 mcg
Calcium	1,000 mg	1,697 mg
Choline	450 mg	591 mg
EPA and DHA	350 mg EPA, 300 mg DHA	115 mg EPA, 120 mg DHA
Fiber	28 g	54 g
Folate/folic acid	600 DFE	1,333 DFE
Iron	27 mg	35 mg
Magnesium	350 to 360 mg	573 mg
Phosphorus	700 mg	2,233 mg
Potassium	4.7 g	4.8 g
Zinc	11 mg	31 mg

TOTAL ENERGY: 2,321 calories

Planning Out Your Meals

As I mentioned in the last chapter, planning out your meals is really the best way to ensure you (and your whole family, for that matter) are eating well. I have included another sample menu here using the recipes in this chapter, so you can see how you can easily put together meals in a way that will give you all of the essential nutrients you and your baby need in this trimester.

As you can see, the total amounts of vitamin D, EPA, and DHA are only about half of the recommended daily amounts. That is because the menu does not include fish, and very few other sources contain these nutrients. Remember, what matters most is your *average* intake of all nutrients over the course of a few days, not your daily intake. On the other hand, if you'd rather fulfill all the nutritional requirements on a daily basis, on days when you don't eat fatty fish, take a supplement that contains EPA, DHA, and vitamin D.

* * *

By now you are more than midway through your pregnancy. The foods and recipe ideas in this chapter have helped you to eat well and also get the critical nutrients that are key during this period of the development of your baby. Now you are in the home stretch! In the next chapter, we will discuss which foods you particularly need during the final phase of your pregnancy, the third trimester.

CHAPTER 6

The Third Trimester

Mama, you're in the home stretch! In just three months, your baby will be out of your belly and in your arms. But from now until delivery, baby will undergo another period of rapid growth (the third trimester is when baby gains the most weight), even though you may already feel like your bump simply cannot get any bigger. Women often report that the last trimester is the hardest one, both physically and psychologically. And understandably so: at this point, you've gained a significant amount of weight and your belly is indeed large, making many of your daily tasks physically hard to accomplish (not to mention the backaches, constipation, hemorrhoids, heartburn, and swelling), and some anxiety about childbirth and labor pains may be really setting in. It is essential that you use all the support systems you have to help you out at this time: your partner, siblings, parents, children, friends, and prenatal care team. On a brighter note, many women in their third trimester have what is called the "nesting" syndrome, experiencing bouts of energy and accomplishing everything they need to get done in preparation for the baby's arrival—so you have something to look forward to besides the birth.

In this chapter, I will discuss some of the best sources to get the key nutrients you need in the last trimester, as well as eating patterns and ways to ensure that your weight stays in check. This is the time when most weight gain occurs, putting you at risk for excessive weight gain. Just as I did in the first and second trimester chapters, I will give an overview of the developmental stages that your baby is undergoing, present a key food for each week, and provide you with some nutritious and easy-to-make recipes to best support your baby's growth and keep your own weight gain within the recommended range.

The third trimester is when your baby grows the most both physically and mentally, acquiring most of its weight and gaining the most brain mass.

In addition, your baby's eyes, teeth, and external genitalia continue to develop and mature until it is born. Because so much growth happens in the last three months, and because this is the time when many vitamins, minerals, and other nutrients are physically transferred to your baby for accumulation, your main mission is to ensure adequate intake of calories and nutrients to provide the proper supply of nourishment your baby needs. And although inadequate intake may not lead to serious developmental issues, your baby may not reach its full growth and development potential as it otherwise would have with good prenatal nutrition.

Now is the time to really stock up on nutrient-packed foods to ensure that your baby has access to all the vitamins and minerals from your diet to build up stores that are adequate and will last until you introduce solid foods. Recipes in this section continue to use a variety of nutrient-rich foods, with a special focus on high-fiber foods that help combat constipation, which is very common in the third trimester. A selection of low-sodium recipes is also provided, which may be of special importance if your doctor has recommended you limit your salt intake due to preeclampsia. Quick-fix meals using store-bought rotisserie chicken and slow cooker recipes are also included as appealing options, because in these final months, being on your feet in the kitchen for long stretches is *not* appealing. Many of the recipes in this section can be prepared in 20 minutes or less, so you have time to get the rest you need (and finish organizing the nursery!).

Heartburn

You may have experienced some heartburn already in your first or second trimester, and if you haven't yet, you're (unfortunately) likely to during the third trimester. Your estrogen and progesterone levels are making your esophageal sphincter muscle more relaxed (it's the muscle at the bottom of your esophagus that prevents the backing up of the stomach's contents into the esophagus); combined with the growing baby and your expanding belly, which is now likely pressing on your stomach, this can lead to heartburn. Also known as acid indigestion, heartburn occurs when the acidic contents of your stomach back up into your esophagus and cause a burning sensation. Studies show that the prevalence of heartburn increases throughout pregnancy, and nearly 72 percent of women experience it in the third trimester, although many (43 percent) also first experience it in the first and/or second trimester. Your risk for pregnancy heartburn is increased by a higher prepregnancy BMI, having heartburn before pregnancy, experiencing nausea and vomiting, gaining more weight during pregnancy, and drinking coffee. However, even though heartburn is not a pleasant thing to deal with, don't be alarmed; it does not appear to adversely affect your baby, and there are ways to manage it.

To reduce your symptoms, try the following:

- Aim for six small, nutrient-dense meals per day instead of three larger ones. Your stomach volume is decreased due to your expanded uterus and ever-growing baby, so consuming smaller meals puts less pressure on your stomach.

- Avoid lying down for one or two hours after a meal.

- Sleep with your head and upper body slightly elevated, to a level higher than your stomach.

- Avoid drinking fluids with your meal. Instead, drink either half an hour before or an hour after a meal.

- Eat lots of fiber-rich foods, every day if possible, to reduce constipation, which means more waste in your lower intestine next to your expanding uterus.

- Wear loose-fitting clothes, especially around your waist.

- Eat slowly and chew your food as thoroughly as you can.

- Avoid spicy and fried foods and foods that you have noticed trigger heartburn. Speak to your doctor about taking an antacid. Tums and similar over-the-counter medications are generally safe to use while pregnant.

- If symptoms persist despite adjusting your diet and taking an over-the-counter antacid, speak to your doctor about other medication options.

It's Time to Ramp Up Your Calories a Little Bit More!

With the accelerated growth of your baby, as well as your increasing blood and body fluid volume, you need extra calories now to support the healthy development of your baby as well as the expansion of your own tissues. You needed 340 additional daily calories in the second trimester, and you need even a bit more during the final one: 450 extra calories per day until your baby is born. Because your nutrient needs are highly increased and because your baby will also start storing some of the nutrients during this trimester for use after birth, it is essential that you "spend" the extra calories wisely. Choosing nutrient-dense foods will ensure adequate nutritional support for your baby and its nutrient stores, as well as provide adequate nutrition for you.

450 CALORIES ────────────────────────────────

What does 450 calories look like? The additional calories that you need in the third trimester are the equivalent of a couple of snacks or even a full meal. However, choose them wisely and try to get the most nutrients for each calorie you consume. An additional 450 calories is equivalent to:

3 ounces of grilled wild salmon, 1 cup of cooked asparagus, 1 medium sweet potato baked in its skin, and 1 cup (8 ounces) of whole milk

1 cup of low-fat yogurt, 1 ounce of walnuts, and 1 large apple

1 ounce of dark chocolate with 70% to 85% cacao solids, 1 cup of raw blueberries, 1 large orange, and 2 slices of low-fat Swiss cheese

1 avocado, 1 medium tomato, and 12 unsalted tortilla chips

Week 26

(Gestational Week 28)

Believe it or not, your baby's first cries may happen this week.

What's Happening?

This week, your baby will finally start opening its eyes (but only a tiny bit). These have been shut since the first trimester. The eyelashes have now finished forming, and the wrinkly skin starts to smooth out a bit because baby is rapidly gaining weight. By the end of week 26, your baby will weigh about 2¼ pounds. Interestingly, while you may have thought that your baby wouldn't cry until delivery time, some research shows that babies can actually cry while still in the womb (who knew?!) as early as 28 weeks of gestation and possibly even earlier. It's not a bad thing (and there's no evidence that a baby is doing this in response to pain), although research is still under way as to why it happens

what to eat when you're pregnant

and what that means. Some scientists believe that through crying and grimacing in the womb, the babies are learning how to communicate with their parents after birth and alert them to their needs. Developmentally, however, it's sort of a big deal, as crying is a complex action that requires a coordinated effort of several motor systems and a negative reaction to a stimulus. Finally, even though your baby still has a full trimester to go, babies born at this time have a 90 percent chance of surviving, and the odds improve with each extra week.

Food of the Week: Coho Salmon

Featured as the food of the week early in the first trimester, salmon is once again the food of the week early in the third trimester. Why? Because it's a true nutrient powerhouse. It has tons of the invaluable vitamins, minerals, and protein that you needed earlier in the pregnancy and are in especially high demand now. Four ounces of cooked coho salmon have 31 g of protein, 0.8 mg of iron, almost 9 mg of niacin, 5 mcg of vitamin B12 (almost double what you need per day!), one-third of your daily vitamin B6 needs (0.63 mg), more than 0.5 g of potassium (516 mg), and half of your daily phosphorus needs (338 mg), as well as smaller amounts of other vitamins and minerals such as calcium, magnesium, zinc, and vitamin A. Most important, salmon has more than double the required daily amount of DHA, with a whopping 745 mg per 4-ounce serving. Brain development is rapid now and on through the rest of the third trimester, and optimal DHA intake is key. Your baby will be absorbing it in the weeks to come, and salmon will be a great source of DHA. If you haven't already, be sure to try the mouthwatering recipe for Maple-Soy Glazed Salmon (page 62) from the first trimester chapter. However, if you don't feel like cooking much these days (oh, my aching back and swollen feet!), treat yourself and your partner to dinner out; many restaurants have coho and other salmon varieties on their menus.

Mom-Safe Sushi Bowl

SERVES 2

This recipe has all the great flavors of sushi without the painstaking rolling or the expense of dining out. Look for pickled ginger in the refrigerated section of Asian markets or near the seafood department of mainstream groceries (it may be labeled gari). You can use ¾ cup of cooked rice instead of the seaweed if you prefer; just skip the first step.

½ cup dried wakame seaweed

4 teaspoons rice vinegar

2 teaspoons soy sauce, plus more for serving

Wasabi paste

1 cucumber, thinly sliced

6 radishes, thinly sliced

6 large cooked shrimp (cooled)

8 ounces cooked wild salmon (cooled)

½ avocado, sliced lengthwise

Sesame seeds (optional)

Pickled ginger

Place the dried wakame in a bowl; cover with cold water and soak for 6 minutes. Drain the wakame well and return it to the bowl.

In another small bowl, combine the rice vinegar, soy sauce, and ¼ teaspoon of wasabi paste and whisk to blend. Add more wasabi if desired. Pour the dressing over the rehydrated wakame and toss to coat. Transfer to a serving bowl.

Arrange the cucumber, radishes, shrimp, salmon, and avocado over the wakame. Sprinkle with sesame seeds and serve with pickled ginger and additional soy sauce and wasabi.

Week 27

(Gestational Week 29)

Your baby's bones have now fully formed.

What's Happening?

This week, the overall structure of your baby's bones has completely formed, even though they are still very soft and will continue to mature until delivery. Baby's eyes are almost fully open and are likely blue (this color will often change after birth). As the womb is getting more and more crowded, your baby is moving somewhat less, although it is doing plenty of stretching, twisting, turning, and kicking.

Food of the Week: Walnuts

Another excellent source of nutrients for your baby's growing brain, and a great food for you to snack on in between meals, walnuts can be easily incorporated

what to eat when you're pregnant

into trail mix, added to a salad, or simply eaten on their own. An ounce of raw walnuts (about 14 walnut halves) has more than the daily dose of essential omega-3 fats (2.6 g), 2 g of fiber, 0.82 mg of iron, and over 13 g of polyunsaturated fatty acids (including omega-3, -6, and -9 fatty acids). However, just like all nuts, walnuts are high in calories, so remember to snack mindfully on this brain food, which has 185 calories in a single ounce. In addition to the recipe below, check out Roasted or Raw Beet Salad (page 60).

Cucumber and Baby Kale Salad with Edamame, Toasted Walnuts, and Mustard Vinaigrette

SERVES 2

Toasting walnuts really brings out their flavor and is worth the few minutes of time and effort it takes. I prefer to toast them in a skillet instead of in the oven, because they are less likely to get burned. You can toast several ounces of walnuts at once if you like and keep extras in a plastic bag to sprinkle on salads.

1 ounce walnuts
1 cup frozen shelled edamame (green soybeans)
¼ cup water
1 teaspoon extra-virgin olive oil
2 teaspoons red wine vinegar
1 teaspoon Dijon mustard
½ teaspoon salt
¼ teaspoon freshly ground black pepper
1 English cucumber, chopped
3 ounces baby kale
¼ cup sliced onion

Place the walnuts in a dry skillet over medium-low heat and toast, stirring frequently, until golden brown spots appear, about 8 minutes. Remove from the skillet and allow to cool in a small bowl.

Place the edamame and water in a microwave-safe bowl and heat on high for 2 minutes. Allow the edamame to sit for 2 minutes, then drain and allow them to cool to room temperature before adding to the salad.

In a large bowl, stir together the olive oil, vinegar, mustard, salt, and pepper. Add the cucumber, kale, onion, and edamame and toss with the dressing, then divide the salad between two plates. Top with the toasted walnuts.

Week 28

(Gestational Week 30)

Wink at me, baby.

What's Happening?

Your baby's eyes started opening a couple of weeks ago; this week baby can finally open them fully and blink. Complete eye functions, such as pupil dilation and contraction, have not fully developed, but will happen in the next few weeks. In addition, your baby's head is now entirely covered by thick hair that has been growing fast since the last trimester. By the end of this week, your baby will weigh nearly 3 pounds, and it will continue to gain more weight as well as start regulating its own body temperature.

Food of the Week: Atlantic Herring or Sardines

A real DHA goldmine, Atlantic herring (aka sardines) is one of the biggest sources of this essential omega-3 fatty acid. A cooked 3-ounce serving will provide you with 940 mg of DHA, as well as about 773 mg of EPA. And the same 3 ounces will give you 20 g of protein, 1.2 mg of iron, more than 11 mcg of vitamin B12, and nearly one-third of your daily recommended intake of vitamin D (4.6 mcg), while also providing you with moderate amounts of vitamins A, E, and B6, and niacin, zinc, potassium, and phosphorus. Pacific herring is another good option in terms of the amount of DHA per serving, but it has slightly less DHA than the Atlantic variety.

Sardines on Crackers

SERVES 2 TO 4

Atlantic herring is commonly canned. This inexpensive seafood is one of the healthiest foods you can eat, and as one of the most sustainable fish choices it is environmentally friendly, too. Look for high-quality sardines canned in olive oil or tomato sauce; avoid the cheap ones canned with sunflower oil.

8 to 12 canned sardines, packed in olive oil or tomato sauce
½ teaspoon white vinegar
2 tablespoons minced red onion
4 whole grain crispbread crackers such as Wasa, Kavli, or Ryvita

Drain the sardines and flake them into a bowl. Add the vinegar and minced onion and stir to combine. Spread the mixture on top of the crackers and serve.

Week 29

(Gestational Week 31)

Your baby is now storing up nutrients on its own.

What's Happening?

Starting this week, your baby will begin to store calcium, iron, phosphorus, and other vitamins and minerals that will help it get through the first six months of life before solid foods are introduced. If you're expecting a girl, her reproductive organs, and more specifically her genitals, will be undergoing a serious developmental surge, becoming much more defined. If you're expecting a boy, his testes will be descending into his scrotum.

Food of the Week: Anchovies

True hoarders of DHA (and other omega-3 fatty acids), anchovies boast a whopping 730 mg in a 2-ounce serving. In addition, anchovies are rich in protein, calcium, potassium, zinc, phosphorus, niacin, and vitamins B12, E, and K. They also have 2.63 mg of iron and contain moderate amounts of magnesium, as well as vitamins D and B6. However, canned anchovies also contain lots of sodium. The same 2-ounce serving, delivering 2.1 g of salt, will put you close to the recommended limit of daily salt intake, which is 2.3 g if you're in generally good health, although recommendations differ, and the more conservative ones recommend consuming only up to 1.5 g per day. It may therefore be a good idea to consume little salt from other sources on days when you eat anchovies, or eat smaller portions (for example, just 1 ounce) over the course of several days. Or (especially if you need to limit your salt intake due to being at higher risk for certain conditions such as preeclampsia) you can soak them in cold water for about 30 minutes and then pat them dry with a paper towel before eating; this will wash away some of the salt and reduce the overall sodium content of these little swimmers. You can buy canned anchovies in most grocery stores, and you can easily add them to a salad or eat them with a slice of bread as a quick snack (as standing while cooking or preparing food may seem not so appealing these days). You could also add anchovies to a pizza or add a teaspoon of anchovy paste to marinara sauce, which adds flavor without overpowering the sauce.

Anchovy, Parsley, and Parmesan Cheese Quiche

SERVES 6

Using phyllo dough for this quiche instead of traditional pastry produces a thin, flaky crust and saves hundreds of calories and dozens of fat grams.

Cooking spray
5 sheets phyllo dough, thawed if frozen
1 (2-ounce) can anchovies packed in oil, drained
½ cup finely chopped onion
4 eggs
½ cup 1% cottage cheese
3 tablespoons chopped parsley (flat leaf or curly)
4 tablespoons grated Parmesan (1 ounce)
Freshly ground black pepper

Preheat the oven to 375°F. Spray a glass or metal pie plate with cooking spray.

Lay a piece of plastic wrap on a countertop and unroll the phyllo dough on top of it. Place one sheet of the phyllo dough in the pie plate, folding back the edges so they do not hang over the edge of the plate. Spray with cooking spray. Add a second sheet of dough, overlapping the first piece, folding the edges back so they do not overhang. Spray with cooking spray. Repeat, coating each sheet with cooking spray, until 5 sheets of dough are layered in the pie plate.

Drain the anchovies and set aside 5 whole pieces; chop the remaining anchovies. In a large mixing bowl, combine the chopped anchovies, onion, eggs, cottage cheese, parsley, 3 tablespoons of the Parmesan cheese, and pepper. Pour the filling into the prepared phyllo crust and place the whole anchovies on top.

Bake for 30 minutes, then sprinkle the remaining 1 tablespoon of Parmesan on top. Bake for 2 minutes more, until the center is solid. Serve warm or at room temperature. Store leftovers in the refrigerator for up to 5 days.

what to eat when you're pregnant

Week 30

(Gestational Week 32)

Just breathe.

What's Happening?

The highlight of the 30th week is that your baby is now starting to practice breathing! This is breathing in utero, during which baby is moving its little diaphragm, even though lung development is not yet complete and will continue all the way up to delivery. However, this practice is preparing your baby for the first gasps of air upon birth, and as you well know, practice makes perfect! In addition, the fine peachlike lanugo hair that has been covering your baby's body for many weeks now is starting to shed (normally, little to none is present at birth). By the end of the week, your baby will weigh close to 3.75 pounds.

Food of the Week: Brown or Wild Rice

Both brown and wild rice are great sources of carbohydrates, for which your needs are significantly increased throughout pregnancy (remember, you should aim for at least 175 g of carbs every day). Importantly, brown and wild rice contain the good carbs—complex carbohydrates—which is the category that most of your carb intake should come from. And they have a lower glycemic index, meaning that they don't cause a sugar rush in your body during digestion, like white flour products or candy bars. In addition, brown and wild rice contain a moderate yet balanced mix of the vitamins and nutrients that you and your baby need. One cup (about 195 g) of medium-grain brown rice has nearly 46 g of carbs, 3.5 g of fiber, over 1 mg of iron, 2.6 mg of niacin, and moderate amounts of protein, calcium, magnesium, phosphorus, potassium, zinc, and vitamin B6. Remember that the absorption of non-heme iron is enhanced by acidic foods and meats, so choose green veggies, fish, poultry, or meat alongside your rice (or have some citrus fruits for dessert afterward; oranges and tangerines are excellent choices). In addition to the recipes below, brown or wild rice goes well with Teriyaki Chicken and Pineapple Skillet (page 121) or Chicken Thighs with Spicy Peanut Sauce (page 83).

Stuffed Portobello Caps with Wild Rice, Cherries, and Pecans

SERVES 4

This light vegetarian dish can be served as a side dish or a meal. You can substitute brown rice and/or dried cranberries in this recipe if you like.

4 large portobello mushroom caps, stems removed (16 ounces)
2 cups cooked wild rice
½ cup dried cherries
½ cup chopped pecans
¾ teaspoon salt
¼ teaspoon freshly ground black pepper
2 eggs

Preheat the oven to 400°F. Line a baking sheet with parchment paper.

Place the mushroom caps on the parchment, gill-side up. In a mixing bowl, combine the rice, cherries, pecans, salt, pepper, and eggs. Stir to blend. Fill the mushroom caps with the rice mixture, mounding up as needed. Bake for 25 minutes, until the filling is dry when lightly touched. Serve warm.

Marinated Wasabi Steak with Brown Rice Pilaf

SERVES 4

Wasabi in the marinade gives this steak a piquant flavor. If you really love the flavor of wasabi, serve extra alongside the steak.

1 tablespoon wasabi paste
1 tablespoon soy sauce
½ teaspoon garlic powder
½ teaspoon ground ginger
1 teaspoon sesame oil or extra-virgin olive oil
1 pound lean steak (such as London broil or top round)
2 cups water
½ teaspoon salt
2 teaspoons extra-virgin olive oil
2 cups instant brown rice (such as Minute brand)
2 cups frozen peas and carrots, thawed
4 tablespoons slivered almonds

Combine the wasabi paste, soy sauce, garlic, ginger, and sesame oil in a resealable plastic bag and mix by kneading the outside of the bag with your hands. Add the steak and seal the bag, removing as much air as possible. Marinate for at least 2 hours and up to 24 hours.

In a pot, bring the water, salt, and olive oil to a boil over high heat. Add the rice, cover the pot, and turn the heat to low. Cook for 5 minutes. Turn off the heat, stir, and replace the cover. Let the rice steam for 5 minutes more, then add the peas, carrots, and almonds and stir. Leave covered on the burner to keep warm.

Preheat a grill. Remove the marinated steak from the bag; discard the bag and remaining marinade. Grill the steak to an internal temperature of 140°F for medium rare, or to your liking. Serve with the rice and vegetables alongside.

Week 31

(Gestational Week 33)

Look at me now.

What's Happening?
Week 31 is another eye-centered one. Your baby has developed the full ability to react to light—its pupils can dilate and constrict—and now is practicing opening and closing its eyes. In addition, the lungs are close to being fully developed, and your baby continues to practice breathing techniques with amniotic fluid, inhaling and exhaling small amounts of it in preparation for doing the same with air at birth. By the end of this week, your baby will weigh more than 4 pounds.

Food of the Week: Kale
This glorified (and justifiably so) leafy green is one that you may be quite familiar with. Its merits lie in the density of nutrients it possesses in a relatively small serving. With the amount of growing, developing, and breathing your baby is now doing, there's no better time than the present to load up on kale. Two cups of kale contain nearly 5 g of fiber, one-fifth of your daily calcium, 2 mg of iron (non-heme), more than 650 mg of potassium, 160 mg of vitamin C, nearly 200 mg of folate, more than 670 mcg of vitamin A, 945 mcg of vitamin K, and moderate amounts of vitamins E and B6, niacin, zinc, phosphorus, and magnesium. A true nutritional powerhouse! Raw kale can be the main

ingredient in a salad (with the right treatment to soften it up a tad), or you can steam it or stir-fry it and enjoy it as a side dish with your main meal. You can even toss some into a blender with fruit to make a green smoothie. Kale has more vitamins A, C, and K than your daily requirement; these are highly beneficial at this time as well as throughout the third trimester. Vitamins A and C help boost your immune system, and vitamin C also helps maintain your skin's elasticity, which is essential for helping to minimize the appearance of stretch marks. In addition, the high amount of vitamin K will help keep your blood vessels strong and healthy (blood volume and supply is highly increased throughout the third trimester) and will ensure proper blood clotting during delivery. Finally, your baby has now developed many visual capacities, and the high amount of vitamin A in kale supports eye development. Because kale contains a few of the fat-soluble vitamins (mostly A and K), you can increase their absorption by adding a splash of healthy fat, such as olive oil, to a kale salad. There are no known downsides to consuming high doses of vitamin K from foods, so do not stress about that. In addition to the recipe below, also check out Roasted or Raw Beet Salad (page 60) and Cucumber and Baby Kale Salad with Edamame, Toasted Walnuts, and Mustard Vinaigrette (page 109).

Sea Salt and Vinegar Kale Chips

SERVES 2 TO 4

Craving a salty, tangy crunch? These will hit the spot. Unlike potato chips or other packaged snacks, these are packed with nutrients and fiber—not unhealthy fats, artificial colors, and preservatives.

1 bunch kale (curly or black kale)
2 teaspoons extra-virgin olive oil
2 tablespoons white vinegar
½ teaspoon coarse sea salt

Preheat the oven to 300°F. Line 2 baking sheets with parchment paper.

Wash the kale, remove the tough stems, and tear into bite-size pieces. Spin in a salad spinner to dry as much as possible. In a large bowl, combine the kale with the olive oil and vinegar. Massage with your hands for 1 to 2 minutes to coat the leaves completely and soften the kale. Spread the kale in a single layer on the prepared sheets, avoiding overlap as much as possible, and sprinkle with sea salt.

Bake the kale for 25 to 30 minutes, until crisp and dry. Store in an airtight container in the refrigerator for up to 5 days.

Week 32

(Gestational Week 34)

Ten fingers, ten nails.

What's Happening?

Your baby's fingernails have been growing fast and are now at the level of its fingertips (you will have to cut them soon after delivery). Just like in the preceding few weeks, your baby may not be moving much due to the cramped living quarters. Pretty much all of its organs, with the exception of the lungs and brain, are now mature. By the end of the week, your baby will weigh about 4½ pounds.

Food of the Week: Acorn Squash

Because your belly has gotten quite large at this point and your uterus has pushed your intestines up a bit (it may feel like they're up to your throat!), not to mention your estrogen-relaxed gut, constipation may be your unwelcome friend this week. High-fiber foods are key throughout the third (as well as the second) trimester, and acorn squash is a great choice, providing you with 6 g of fiber per cup. In addition, it has nearly 30 g of protein, almost 2 mg of iron, and nearly 900 mg of potassium (that's close to one-quarter of your daily needs), and also provides some calcium, magnesium, and phosphorus, as well as vitamins C and B6. In addition to the recipe below, check out Sweet Stuffed Winter Squash with Coconut and Yogurt (page 97) from week 23.

Roast Pork Tenderloin with Apples, Squash, and Golden Raisins

SERVES 2 TO 4

Pork tenderloin is not only one of the leanest cuts of pork but also the most versatile. It can be prepared in about 30 minutes, far less time than roasting a whole chicken, for example. Like other cuts of pork, the tenderloin is delicious paired with fruits and warm spices, as in this recipe.

1 pork tenderloin
2 to 3 teaspoons prepared Dijon mustard
Salt and freshly ground black pepper

Onion powder

Garlic powder

1 teaspoon extra-virgin olive oil

¾ cup peeled, chopped acorn or butternut squash

1 firm sweet apple, cored and chopped

2 teaspoons apple cider vinegar

⅛ teaspoon salt

⅛ teaspoon ground cinnamon

⅛ teaspoon nutmeg

1 tablespoon golden raisins

1 tablespoon water

Preheat the oven to 425°F. Line a baking dish with foil.

Rub the entire surface of the pork with the mustard and season all sides with a light sprinkling of salt, pepper, onion powder, and garlic powder. Place on the prepared pan and bake for 25 minutes, until an instant-read thermometer reads 150°F in the thickest part. Allow the pork to rest for 10 minutes before slicing.

Meanwhile, heat the oil in a large skillet over medium heat. Add the squash and apple and cook for 10 minutes, stirring occasionally. Add the vinegar, salt, cinnamon, and nutmeg and stir to blend. Stir in the raisins and water, cover, and reduce the heat to very low. Cook for 10 minutes, then keep warm until ready to serve.

Serve the sliced pork topped with the apple and squash mixture.

Week 33

(Gestational Week 35)

Getting ready for its grand entrance, baby is now head down!

What's Happening?

The lanugo hair is almost entirely gone now; the creamy vernix is still there and is actually getting a bit thicker now, continuing to protect your baby's delicate skin. Baby's little lungs have almost finished developing at this point, and baby is continuing to diligently practice the breathing routine. If baby hasn't already turned into its birth position (head down), that will likely happen this week.

Food of the Week: Collard Greens

Another nutrient-rich leafy green somewhat similar to kale, collards are simply packed with the nutrients you need at this time. Collards are usually available in supermarkets year-round, but if you can't get them fresh, frozen ones are just as good (as they're picked at their prime and frozen immediately, which preserves all the nutrients). One cup (about 190 g) of cooked collards is rich in fiber and calcium (containing about one-quarter of your daily needs for both) and has more than 2 mg of iron and more than one-third of your daily dose of vitamin C, which will help your body absorb the non-heme iron. In addition, collards are rich in vitamin A and beta-carotene, provide half of your daily manganese, have tons of vitamin K (that cup of cooked collards has more than 770 mcg of vitamin K), and are moderately good sources of choline, pantothenic acid, zinc, potassium, phosphorus, and magnesium. You can easily add collards, either fresh or cooked, as a side to almost any main dish, and especially to meat, poultry, and fish entrées. The iron present in meat will further increase the amount you absorb from the collards, upping your overall iron stores at this time.

Garlicky Mixed Beans and Collard Greens

SERVES 4

Serve this side dish with rotisserie chicken or spoon it over cooked quinoa for a meatless entrée that's ready in a flash. The ingredients are shelf-stable, too.

1 (10-ounce) box frozen collard greens (chopped) or
    3½ cups chopped fresh
1 (15-ounce) can mixed beans
½ cup tomato sauce or tomato-based pasta sauce
½ teaspoon garlic powder
½ teaspoon onion powder
1 tablespoon hot sauce (such as Frank's Red Hot)

In a skillet over medium-low heat, combine all of the ingredients. Cook for 10 minutes, until warmed through, then serve.

Week 34

(Gestational Week 36)

Baby is putting on the pounds.

What's Happening?

This week, your baby will get serious about weight gain and start putting on the pounds faster than ever, with a steady ½ pound per week until delivery (so with every pound that you gain, about half is going to the baby). I know that it may seem like there's literally no way you could gain another ounce, but remember that a lot of what you gain is actually what your baby is gaining. At the end of week 34, it will be about 6 pounds.

Food of the Week: Chicken

Chicken is the second of two foods that are featured twice as foods of the week (salmon was the first). That's because it's simply perfect for you and your baby at this time, as well as throughout the third trimester. Half of a chicken breast (without skin) has 27 g of protein, nearly 1 mg of iron, 12 mg of niacin, 0.3 mcg of vitamin B12, over ½ mg of vitamin B6, and moderate amounts of phosphorus, potassium, and zinc. Remember to always remove the skin regardless of what part of the chicken you're eating because it contains a lot of cholesterol and is high in animal fat, neither of which you need.

To make sure you get all the nutrients you need, I've included four delicious recipes. In addition, you should revisit the recipe for Rotisserie Chicken with Apricot Quinoa over Spinach (page 89) from week 18, as well as the three chicken recipes from week 15 starting on page 82.

Slow Cooker BBQ-Salsa Chicken

SERVES 6

Use this versatile shredded chicken to top a green salad or fill whole wheat tortillas, along with lettuce and grated cheese, for an easy dinner. You can also substitute a lean beef roast for a beef version.

2 pounds skinless boneless chicken breast (or skinless boneless thighs)
⅓ cup bottled barbecue sauce
½ cup bottled salsa

Place the chicken in a slow cooker and pour the barbecue sauce and salsa over the top. Cook on low heat for 6 hours, then remove and shred with two forks to serve.

Rotisserie Chicken with Cajun Corn and Zucchini

SERVES 2

Most grocery stores have rotisserie chickens ready to grab for a convenient healthy meal option. Here's an easy meal idea that you can pull together in just 10 minutes!

1 tablespoon extra-virgin olive oil
1 large zucchini, cut into approximately 1-inch cubes
2 cups frozen corn kernels
1 tablespoon Cajun seasoning blend (or more to taste)
½ teaspoon lime juice
1 rotisserie chicken

Heat the oil in a large nonstick skillet over medium heat. Add the zucchini and corn, cover, and cook for 5 minutes. Add the Cajun seasoning and lime juice, and continue to cook, uncovered, until the zucchini reaches its desired tenderness.

Meanwhile, remove the skin from the chicken and put 4 ounces of cooked meat onto each of two plates. (Refrigerate the leftover chicken for another meal.) Keep the plates warm in the oven set to the lowest temperature, if needed.

Serve the vegetables alongside the chicken.

Teriyaki Chicken and Pineapple Skillet

SERVES 2

This low-fat one-skillet meal makes an easy dinner for two, with protein, vegetables, and fruit all in one course. Serve with steamed broccoli for a lower-carbohydrate option or rice for a more substantial dinner.

2 chicken breasts
4 slices canned pineapple rings
Salt and freshly ground black pepper
1 teaspoon extra-virgin olive oil
½ yellow onion, chopped
1 green bell pepper, cored, seeded, and chopped
1 red, orange, or yellow bell pepper, cored, seeded, and chopped

½ cup sliced mushrooms

2 cloves garlic, crushed

3 tablespoons teriyaki sauce

2 tablespoons water

Use a paring knife to cut a pocket into the center of each chicken breast. Tuck 1 pineapple ring into each pocket (cut the ring in half if necessary). Secure the pineapple in place with toothpicks and lightly season the outside of the chicken on both sides with salt and pepper.

Heat the oil in a nonstick skillet over medium-high heat. Add the chicken and cook for 4 minutes per side, until golden brown. Reduce the heat to low and add the onion, peppers, mushrooms, garlic, teriyaki sauce, the remaining 2 pineapple rings, and the water. Break up the pineapple rings with a wooden spoon or spatula. Cover and cook for 15 minutes. Remove the lid and allow the sauce to bubble and thicken (if necessary) before turning off the heat. To serve, divide the chicken and vegetables between two plates.

Kickin' Chicken Scallopini

SERVES 2 TO 4

Many grocery stores sell thinly sliced raw chicken breast, which cooks in much less time than a full breast. Turkey breast cutlets thinly sliced in the same way work beautifully in this recipe as well. Steamed vegetables or salad round out the meal.

1 pound thinly sliced boneless skinless chicken breast

2 teaspoons hot sauce (such as Frank's Red Hot)

2 tablespoons ground flaxseed

2 tablespoons almond flour

2 tablespoons dried minced onion

½ teaspoon salt

¼ teaspoon freshly ground black pepper

¼ teaspoon cayenne

Preheat the oven to 400°F. Line a baking sheet with foil or parchment.

Place the chicken in a bowl and add the hot sauce, stirring to coat all pieces. Combine the flaxseed, almond flour, onion, salt, pepper, and cayenne in a small bowl, then spread on a rimmed plate. One at a time, lift the chicken slices, allowing any excess sauce to drip off, and press each side into the coating. Place on the baking sheet in a single layer.

Bake for 15 minutes and serve hot.

(Gestational Week 37)

Congratulations! Your baby is now officially full-term.

What's Happening?

All of your baby's organs are fully formed now and ready to function on their own. This week, your baby is considered full-term (babies born before the 35th week are considered preterm) and weighs about 6½ pounds. Positioned head down in your pelvis, your baby is prepared for delivery and can't wait to meet mommy and the rest of the world! You may or may not be gaining more weight at this time, but if you aren't, don't worry. It is perfectly normal (and quite common) for women to stop gaining weight in the last month of pregnancy, often due to the stomach being squished and not being able to eat a whole lot, as your baby is taking up the available space. However, you may also continue to gain weight, which is normal as well. Either way, continue to choose nutrient-dense (not calorie-dense) foods and keep to a well-balanced diet, just as you have up to this point, especially if you're close to or over your total recommended gestational weight gain.

Food of the Week: Carrots

As you're nearing your due date, you may be feeling pretty full even from small amounts of food. Your stomach has been forced to decrease in size and change shape due to the expanded uterus that seems to have completely taken over your body. However, you still need to nourish yourself and your baby, and choosing small, nutrient-dense snacks instead of full meals may be your best bet. Carrots are a perfect choice, offering plenty of nutrients and not too many calories, and they can be consumed as a light snack so as not to overwhelm your stomach. Raw baby carrots may be particularly practical, as you can carry them in a resealable bag or a small container and snack on them when you feel like it. One serving (about 85 g) contains nearly 0.8 mg of iron and over 200 mg of potassium, has a ton of vitamin A (586 mcg, more than two-thirds of what you need per day), vitamin K (8 mcg), and a little bit of fiber (2.5 g), while containing a mere 30 calories, so feel free to indulge as much (or as little) as you want. In addition to the recipe below, check out Marinated Wasabi Steak with Brown Rice Pilaf (page 114).

Carrot, Cashew, and Ginger Soup

SERVES 2

Many women report that ginger helps settle a queasy stomach, and this smooth soup is tasty hot or cold. It's a lovely orange color and packed with vitamin A.

2 cups chicken or vegetable broth
2 large carrots, sliced
1 ounce (¼ cup) raw unsalted cashews
½ to 1 cup water or additional broth
⅛ teaspoon ground ginger (more if desired)

In a saucepan over high heat, bring the broth to a boil. Add the carrots and boil for 5 to 6 minutes, until soft. Transfer the broth and carrots to a blender and add the cashews. Secure the lid and process on the highest speed until completely smooth. (If your blender lid has a central cap that can be removed, remove it and drape a dishtowel over the top so steam can escape while processing.)

Pour the soup back into the saucepan and heat over medium heat until the soup begins to simmer and thickens slightly. Use ½ cup of water to rinse out the blender and pour that into the pot; add more water or broth to achieve your desired soup consistency.

Stir in the ginger and serve hot.

Week 36

(Gestational Week 38)

Almost there.

What's Happening?

Your baby's brain and nervous systems, even though fully formed, continue to mature. Baby's toenails have grown all the way to the tips of its toes. The vernix coating is starting to disappear now, although some might still be present at the time of birth. Most, if not all of the lanugo hair is now gone. Your baby weighs close to 7 pounds at the end of week 36. If you don't feel like eating large amounts of food these days, opt for snack-size foods six (or even more) times per day.

Food of the Week: Green Beans

Nutritionally quite similar to baby carrots, green beans are another great food for you to focus on now, especially if you're having trouble eating larger quantities of food (or normal quantities, which seem large). One cup (about 100 g) of raw green beans have more than 1 mg of iron, 12 mg of vitamin C, more than 14 mcg of vitamin K (remember, it's involved in proper blood clotting, which is important as you get closer to your delivery date), and moderate amounts of many other vitamins and minerals (folate, vitamin B6, zinc, potassium) and fiber (2.7 g). As with the baby carrots, you can keep a small container of fresh raw beans in your bag and snack away whenever you feel like it. In addition, you can eat them as a side dish, or enjoy a green bean salad for lunch.

Green Beans and Peppers with Dill

SERVES 2

Trimmed green beans cost just a little more than untrimmed ones, but can make dinner prep much faster. This recipe gets plenty of flavor from combining fresh dill, olive oil, garlic, and lemon, so even with no salt, it's anything but bland.

1 (12-ounce) bag trimmed green beans
½ yellow onion, sliced
1 red pepper, cored, seeded, and sliced
¼ cup chopped fresh dill
2 teaspoons extra-virgin olive oil
Garlic powder
Freshly ground black pepper
¼ lemon

Preheat the oven to 425°F. Line a baking sheet with foil.

In a large mixing bowl, combine the green beans, onion, red pepper, dill, and olive oil and toss to coat. Spread on the baking sheet and sprinkle lightly with the garlic powder and black pepper. Bake for 35 minutes, then remove from the oven and squeeze the lemon juice over the vegetables, tossing gently to mix. Serve warm.

Lemon Pepper Sole with Steamed Veggies

This low-sodium dinner takes only about 15 minutes to prepare, which is perfect for when you don't want to be on your feet for long. Serve with wild or brown rice.

1 pound trimmed green beans
½ cup water
1 medium zucchini, chopped
½ cup diced tomatoes (fresh or no-salt-added canned), drained
Pinch of red pepper flakes (optional)
1 pound fresh sole fillet
Salt-free lemon pepper seasoning
2 teaspoons butter
½ lemon, cut into 4 wedges

Preheat the broiler to high. Line a baking sheet with foil.

In a large skillet over medium heat, combine the green beans and water. Cover and bring to a boil, then lower the heat and steam for 4 minutes. Add the zucchini, cover, and steam for 4 minutes more. Drain off any remaining water and add the tomatoes to the skillet. Gently stir, sprinkle with red pepper flakes, then turn the heat down to low.

Place the sole on the baking sheet and sprinkle evenly with lemon pepper. Cut the butter into small pieces and distribute evenly over the fish. Broil for 6 minutes or until the thickest part flakes easily with a fork. Squeeze the juice from 2 of the lemon wedges over the fish. Serve the fish alongside the vegetables with 1 of the remaining lemon wedges on each plate.

Week 37

(Gestational Week 39)

Any day now.

What's Happening?

You're almost done with your pregnancy! You may deliver this week (or have already delivered), or it may still be another week or two until you go into labor. As your doctor may have told you already, delivering anywhere from week 38 to 42 is normal (and can vary even beyond that in some cases). Either way, your baby is fully developed and ready to come out. You may still be gaining some weight at this time, although most women no longer do. Your baby, however, continues putting on some extra ounces and will continue to do so until delivery. At the end of this week, baby is likely a little over 7 pounds.

Food of the Week: Chickpeas

One of my personal favorite foods, chickpeas will super-nourish you and your baby during the final days, ensuring that both of you are in top-notch nutritional shape at delivery time. One cup of cooked chickpeas will provide you with nearly 15 g of protein, 45 g of complex carbohydrate, 12.5 g of fiber, and nearly 5 (yes, 5) mg of iron! Because your baby continues to store iron until the cord is cut shortly after birth, extra iron at this time will boost stores (just remember to eat the chickpeas with something acidic to increase the non-heme iron absorption). In addition, you will get plenty of folate (282 mcg), potassium (480 mg), selenium (6 mcg), manganese (1.7 mg), and some calcium, magnesium, phosphorus, zinc, and vitamin K.

Slow Cooker Pasta Sauce with Roasted Red Peppers, Artichoke Hearts, and Chickpeas

SERVES 4

This recipe represents low-effort, family-friendly cooking at its best. All you need are four pantry items and some whole grain pasta to have a delicious meal. If you like, you can add a pound of cubed pork, beef, or chicken to the slow cooker to boost the protein and B12 content of your meal.

1 (24-ounce) jar tomato-basil pasta sauce
1 (19-ounce) can chickpeas, drained and rinsed
1 (16-ounce) jar roasted red peppers, drained and cut into pieces
1 (6-ounce) jar quartered, marinated artichoke hearts, drained

Combine all of the ingredients in a slow cooker on low heat and cook for 4 hours. Serve over cooked whole wheat pasta or spaghetti squash.

Slow Cooker Indian Spiced Chickpeas

SERVES 4 AS A SIDE DISH, 2 AS A MAIN DISH

Learning to delegate can help you get it all done. For example, let your slow cooker do the work when you've got a busy day. This vegetarian entrée can stand alone as a stew or be scooped up with whole wheat flatbreads.

1 (14-ounce) can diced tomatoes
1 (19-ounce) can chickpeas, drained and rinsed
½ tablespoon garam masala
1 tablespoon curry powder
1 onion (yellow or red), chopped
⅛ teaspoon cayenne pepper (optional)
Fresh cilantro, chopped

Combine the tomatoes, chickpeas, garam masala, curry powder, onion, and cayenne in a slow cooker and stir. Cover and cook for 4 hours on low heat. Serve garnished with the cilantro.

Week 38

(Gestational Week 40)

Oh, baby!

What's Happening?

Congratulations! This is (likely) your last week of pregnancy, and your baby is now due any minute. However, don't stress out if your estimated due date comes and goes uneventfully. Only 5 percent of all women give birth on their estimated due date, and again, most babies are born between weeks 38 and 42, a 4-week range (healthy babies come at different gestational ages and in different sizes). By the end of this week, whether out of the belly or not, your baby will be about 7½ pounds.

Food of the Week: Mango

To finish your pregnancy on a sweet note, mango is the food for this final week. In addition to being delicious, a cup of this fresh fruit will provide you with plenty of carbs, carotene, and vitamin C (remember, vitamin C boosts your skin's elasticity, which is important even in the final days of pregnancy), with smaller amounts of vitamin K, choline, folate, selenium, potassium, and fiber. Enjoy it as a quick snack, part of a dish, or even a dessert.

Shrimp and Mango Kabobs

SERVES 2

Frozen cooked shrimp is a great item to keep on hand for an easy, quick dinner. This recipe combines sweet mango, creamy avocado, and fresh lime and cilantro into a delightful meal.

12 ounces frozen precooked shrimp
1 mango
1 pint grape or cherry tomatoes
½ cup chopped cilantro
1 avocado, chopped
1 lime, cut in half

Thaw the frozen shrimp in a colander under running water. Cut the mango into 1-inch cubes, discarding the peel and seed. Thread one shrimp, one tomato, and one mango cube onto a skewer, and continue this pattern until the skewer is full. Continue with another skewer to use up all the shrimp (you may have leftover tomatoes).

To make a salsa, chop the leftover mango cubes finely and mix with the cilantro and avocado in a bowl. Add the juice from the ½ lime and stir gently.

Preheat an indoor grill. Cook the skewers on the grill for 5 minutes, or until the tomatoes and mango are tender. Divide the skewers between two plates and squeeze the remaining ½ lime over the kabobs. Serve with the avocado-mango salsa.

Planning Out Your Meals

As I did in the first two trimesters, I have created another sample menu using the recipes in this chapter, so you can see how you can easily put together meals in a way that will deliver all of the essential nutrients that you and your baby need during the third trimester.

A balanced diet composed of commonly eaten foods can provide you with all the nutrients you need. In addition, consuming fortified foods—especially

One-Day Sample Menu for the Third Trimester

Breakfast	¾ cup fortified breakfast cereal 1 cup fresh mango, blueberries, and strawberries 1 cup plain, low-fat yogurt
Snack	Cucumber and Baby Kale Salad (page 109)
Lunch	Slow Cooker Indian Spiced Chickpeas (page 128) 3 ounces cooked Atlantic herring 1 teaspoon olive oil 2 cups fresh collard greens, 1 roasted carrot
Snack	1 piece apple pie 1 cup orange juice (fortified with vitamin D and calcium)
Dinner	Rotisserie Chicken with Cajun Corn and Zucchini (page 121) ½ cup brown rice 1 cup sliced fresh pear
Snack	1 open-faced avocado sandwich (1 piece whole wheat toast, ½ avocado, 2 tablespoons hummus, 1 ounce American cheese, and fresh basil leaves) 1 cup skim milk (fortified with vitamins A and D)

Nutrient	Amount Needed Per Day	Provided by Menu
Carbohydrate	175 g	304 g
Protein	1.1 g per kg body weight	127 g
Fat	20% to 35% of total daily calories	93.5 g
Vitamin A	770 mcg RAE/2,565 IU	1,536 mcg RAE
Vitamin B6	1.9 mg	4.9 mg
Vitamin B12	2.6 mcg	20.4 mcg
Vitamin C	85 mg	343 mg
Vitamin D	600 IU (15 mcg)	524 IU
Vitamin K	90 mcg	735 mcg
Calcium	1,000 mg	2,011 mg
Choline	450 mg	469 mg
EPA and DHA	350 mg EPA, 300 mg DHA	775 mg EPA, 939 mg DHA
Fiber	28 g	53.2 g
Folate/folic acid	600 DFE	1,598 DFE
Iron	27 mg	31.5 mg
Magnesium	350 to 360 mg	609 mg
Phosphorus	700 mg	2,496 mg
Potassium	4.7 g	5.6 g
Zinc	11 mg	28.7 mg

TOTAL ENERGY: 2,443 calories

what to eat when you're pregnant

on days when you may not be consuming enough foods with vitamin D, iron, EPA and DHA, or calcium—can fill in the gaps in case you're not getting the needed amount from your diet or are not taking a supplement.

Finally, don't forget to relax. You've done an amazing job, mama, and are about to start a whole new chapter of life with your incredible—and properly nourished—little bundle of joy!

* * *

Congratulations, you made it! You may very well be reading these words while holding your sleepy newborn. In this chapter, we reviewed the key nutrients you should strive to consume in the final weeks of your pregnancy. Next, we will discuss how you can avoid craving pitfalls and discuss other ways in which you can keep your healthy eating plan on track.

PART III

How to Eat Well during and after Pregnancy

CHAPTER 7

My Hormones Made Me Eat It! How to Avoid Using Food to Feel Better

Eating well isn't always as easy as it should be, especially when you are expecting. Part II of this book gave you an overview of the nutrients you and your baby need, and recipes containing the foods you can eat to get them. But all of your good intentions and knowledge can go right out the window when cravings and emotional eating begin.

Much of our pregnancy-related eating can be blamed on hormones. As women, we have been living with monthly hormonal swings for years, but during pregnancy these mood swings and feelings can be exaggerated, and sometimes this causes us to crave foods or to eat foods to soothe ourselves.

Hormones aren't all bad. They are the invisible guides of pregnancy that help our bodies know what to do to grow a baby. But in addition to the emotional rides they are so frequently known to fuel, hormones are the masterminds behind increased food cravings and reduced feelings of satiety (feeling full). Our hormones help us want those extra calories that are needed in the second and third trimesters, but they can also lead us down the path of eating too much, eating the wrong things, and eating for the wrong reasons.

This chapter is meant to introduce you to the major hormones underlying your urges to eat during pregnancy and provides suggestions to help you recognize and avoid craving traps. Knowing how to cope with cravings and emotions that may trigger overeating will prevent you from self-soothing with food. This is especially important because overeating may not only increase your odds of excess weight gain during pregnancy but also (as we discussed in chapter 2) alter your baby's brain circuits that control appetite and promote early-onset obesity as well as other problems.

A Crash Course on Hormones

There are many hormones that regulate different functions in our bodies, and many are critical during pregnancy. Here is a quick summary of a few that are important when thinking about what we eat—and why.

Estrogen

When you are not pregnant, estrogen decreases appetite and food intake by inhibiting the activity of neurons and other molecules that normally make you hungry and by stimulating the molecules that tell you, "I'm full." In fact, the satiating effect of estrogen at different times of a woman's menstrual cycle is thought to be one of the reasons why women's appetites fluctuate on a monthly basis.

During pregnancy, estrogen is involved in maintaining additional functions, including breast enlargement (and the accompanying tenderness) and changes in the womb to prepare for the developing baby. Blood estrogen levels rise during pregnancy, peak at around 40 weeks of gestational age, and rapidly decline after delivery. At this point, you may be wondering: *If estrogen reduces appetite and levels rise during pregnancy, why don't I want to eat* less *during pregnancy?* Read on to find out!

GENDER NEUTRAL ─────────────────────────────

A woman's estrogen levels are the same whether she is carrying a male or a female baby.

Progesterone

Like estrogen, progesterone plays a significant role in eating habits during parts of the menstrual cycle. Unlike estrogen, progesterone stimulates appetite and promotes weight gain—but, importantly, *only* in the presence of estrogen. While estrogen may reduce food intake when its levels are high, progesterone's effect on stimulating hunger overrides the normal influence of estrogen alone. This is thought to be why women tend to eat more during the luteal phase of the menstrual cycle (which spans from the day you ovulate to the day you get your next period) than during any other phase.

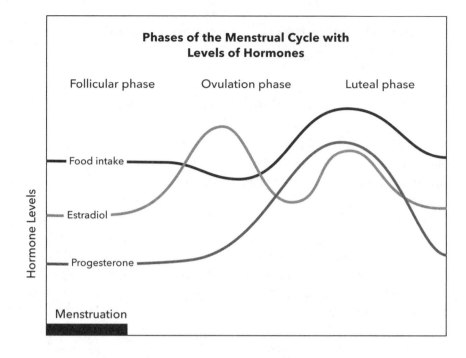

Phases of the Menstrual Cycle with Levels of Hormones

Follicular phase   Ovulation phase   Luteal phase

Hormone Levels

Food intake

Estradiol

Progesterone

Menstruation

During pregnancy, progesterone is responsible for building up the lining of the uterus, effectively establishing the placenta and preventing early uterine contractions. Interestingly, humans secrete much larger amounts of progesterone during gestation than other mammals, peaking around 300 mg per day at term; this is ten times the amount of progesterone than is normally secreted at its greatest concentration during any menstrual cycle. This dramatic rise in progesterone levels throughout pregnancy, coupled with greater levels of estrogen, is one of the primary reasons why your cravings for calorically rich foods may seem almost unbearable during the later stages of pregnancy.

I'M HAVING A GIRL, SO WHY CARE ABOUT TESTOSTERONE? —

Women as well as men secrete testosterone, and it is an influential hormone during pregnancy, even if you are having a baby girl. It rises mildly throughout pregnancy in the bloodstream and drops off in the postpartum period. Testosterone increases appetite and food intake (including binge-eating behaviors) by affecting brain mechanisms, and it also increases the accumulation of abdominal fat.

Leptin

Leptin does not have much *direct* association with pregnancy but is involved in controlling our eating habits throughout our entire lives. Leptin is the primary hormone that tells you that you're full. It is released by adipose (or fat) cells, particularly after a meal, and acts on the hypothalamus—a key part of the brain involved in regulating appetite and food intake. In many obese and overweight people, a phenomenon occurs in which the brain becomes resistant to the effects of leptin. In other words, despite the presence of this hormone, such individuals will not feel full (or as full) after a meal and may therefore continue to eat. People who experience this reduced satiated feeling are said to have *leptin resistance*. Keep this in mind as you read the following section.

Prolactin and Human Placental Lactogen

You may be able to guess the best-known function of the hormone prolactin: producing milk! Prolactin is produced by the pituitary gland in the brain and increases the number of cells in the breasts that produce milk. Prolactin's blood concentration at term, which is approximately 207 ng/mL (compared to a normal 10 ng/mL in nonpregnant premenopausal women), clearly demonstrates its importance in milk production immediately after delivery. These levels remain elevated until nursing ceases. So why are we talking about this hormone when its primary function appears to occur during lactation? It also has a lesser-known role in influencing appetite.

During pregnancy and lactation, prolactin and human placental lactogen (hPL), which is released by the developing baby, both increase food intake and appetite through their induction of *leptin resistance*. Studies in animals demonstrate that prolactin and hPL cause leptin resistance via actions in the hypothalamus, where they weaken the signaling in your brain that should normally reduce appetite. Instead, they *increase* your appetite, leading to strong urges to overeat. In other words, prolactin and hPL (which are present in high concentrations only during pregnancy) reduce your feelings of fullness, meaning that you may feel hungrier than usual and frequently crave food.

Before moving on to strategies that can be helpful for avoiding overeating due to these hormone-induced urges, it is important to remember that it is the combination of *all* of these hormones throughout pregnancy that influences your feelings of hunger and cravings. Remember, we have evolved this way to ensure appropriate weight gain during pregnancy to support the growth of our babies before and after birth. However, this is certainly not an invitation to completely give in to these cravings (as we discussed in chapter 2). The following sections are tailored to help you navigate the world of cravings while still maintaining a healthy diet.

Am I Really Hungry?

This is the million-dollar question. Cravings are natural, and sometimes they are our body's way of letting us know that we need to eat something. However, cravings can also be triggered by stress, anxiety, or even the modern food environment. (Ever suddenly felt like getting a Frappuccino after walking past a Starbucks? That's no coincidence—that's the advertisement triggering a craving.) So it is important when these cravings pop up to ask yourself whether you are actually hungry. For example, is this a biologically driven craving for food because I am hungry? Or am I seeking out the food for some other reason? Typically, when hunger-driven cravings occur, they are not for specific items (like ice cream), but rather for food groups (such as meat). So if you are craving Rocky Road Häagen-Dazs, you may need to put on the brakes and think about *why* you want it before you give in.

Techniques to Avoid Craving Traps

Considering the number of hormones involved in pregnancy that influence our appetite, it is no wonder we often hear about uncontrollable cravings and late-night trips by attentive partners to the grocery store. Luckily, there are some ways to handle cravings strategically if and when they emerge. With these techniques stowed away in your mind for future use, you won't be caught off guard and defenseless. Instead, you will have strategies in your arsenal to help you cope more confidently with cravings without compromising your health and weight gain goals.

Before going into the specifics of how to deal with cravings, let's briefly discuss the common types of food cravings that may emerge. A recent look at Google searches revealed that pregnant women appear to crave similar things regardless of where in the world they live, whether it be in the United States or India. In the United States, the top search is for "craving *ice* (but not ice cream!) during pregnancy," followed by searches for salt, sweets, fruit, and spicy foods. Additionally, a study of more than 100 pregnant women, of whom 80 percent reported some food cravings when first studied at around 16 to 20 weeks of gestation, found that pregnant women tend to crave sweet (for example, candy, chocolate, cookies, frozen desserts, fruits, fruit juices, soda, sweetened milks, and yogurts) and savory (for example, French fries, meats, pizza, and seafood) foods most. Notably, while cravings for sweets tended to peak at 24 to 28 weeks of pregnancy (accompanied by increased fruit and fruit juice intake), food cravings in general appeared to decrease over the course of pregnancy. Since frequently eating high-calorie desserts and treats can add up to excess weight gain, I've made sure to include low-sugar dessert recipes in Part II to keep your sweet tooth satisfied at a reasonable calorie level. Using fruit and low-sugar desserts to address your cravings can also help control blood sugar, which is especially important if you've developed impaired glucose tolerance or gestational diabetes.

THAT IRRESISTIBLE CRAVING ───────────────────────────

What is the craziest pregnancy craving you have heard of? It doesn't have to be food. A friend told me that when she was pregnant with her first child she craved the smell of Home Depot!

Expect the Best, Prepare for the Worst

When intense hunger strikes, health is usually not our first priority; instead, we typically end up eating what's most conveniently available. Thus the first step to avoid eating (and overeating) unhealthy foods, such as those high in added fats and sugars (and generally of little nutritional value), is to plan ahead. Before you find yourself famished or a craving has set in, prepare by having healthy "quick fixes" ready in your home, or even in your bag, at all times. Also, try to identify what aspect of a food or drink you are craving when you feel the urge for something. Are you craving the crunchiness of the food? The sweetness? Maybe the cold, bubbly taste of a soda? By identifying exactly *what* it is you are craving, you can start to brainstorm healthier alternatives that will satisfy your urge without compromising your goals. For instance, if it's the crunch you really want, grab a handful of carrots or almonds when you sit down to watch something on Netflix, instead of going for the bag of chips. If it's the bubbly taste (carbonation), try flavored seltzer water. If it's the sweet taste, try to keep your favorite fruits in the house. Although some fruits can contain a lot of sugar, especially dried fruits, they can also be a good source of nutrients such as antioxidants and fiber, making them healthier than soda, cake, cookies, or candy.

Want a healthy quick fix to stave off a sugar craving, but don't like the looks (or the price) of those processed "health" bars? Try making your own energy bars. They are easy, and you can customize them to your liking. Grab your food processor, and start off with a base of one or two handfuls of dried apricots and approximately 8 ounces of dates (try to get dates without added sugar—check the label). Then add in a handful of cashews (or other nuts that you like) and a few squirts of honey. Process for a few minutes, and a ball will form (you may need to add a bit more honey if you have a lot of nuts in there). Press flat with waxed paper into a square baking pan, and then pop it in the freezer. In 30 minutes, you can cut them into bite-size bars and store in plastic bags. These are easy snacks to grab on your way out the door, and because they are homemade, you know what is in them. You can experiment with adding cacao powder, dried cranberries, or whatever else you like.

It Takes a Village

Just as social pressure to "eat for two" or indulge in bottomless pints of ice cream can be persuasive, social support can be an extremely powerful tool in helping us eat foods packed with nutrition during pregnancy. In an effort to show their affection, some partners may buy or make their pregnant loved ones unhealthy foods without realizing this gesture may actually be *too* sweet. Tell your spouse, family, friends, and even coworkers that you hope to stay in good shape and maintain a healthy diet throughout your pregnancy. This way, baked goods won't be forced on you every time you turn around at work, and you and your spouse can prepare and enjoy meals together that will promote the healthy development of your baby. Also, if you make your goals known, it may be easier to solicit help along the way if you find yourself struggling to stay on track.

Get a Good Night's Rest . . .
and Don't Sweat the Small Stuff

There is a considerable amount of research that suggests a strong link between sleep and appetite, and pregnant women are no exception. In fact, fatigue has been linked to increased caloric intake in general, increased consumption of carbohydrates, fats, and proteins, as well as decreased folate intake during pregnancy, highlighting the importance of getting an adequate amount of rest. Additionally, it appears that stress levels may influence what we eat, as stress has been associated with increased consumption of breads, fats, oils, sweets, and snacks during pregnancy. Therefore, try to prevent sources of stress whenever possible. I know, that is often easier said than done, but there *are* things you can do.

If you feel stressed and find yourself headed for the pantry, experiment with some nonfood activities first to help you clear your mind and relax, such as:

- Going for a walk
- Calling a friend or family member
- Listening to music
- Meditating
- Watching your favorite show
- Reading

If that doesn't work, try plan B: Choose healthy, low-calorie snacks that you can safely munch on when stressed, such as celery sticks or baby carrots, or just about any other vegetable or fruit. That way, even if you do resort to eating when under stress, you'll be getting plenty of vitamins and healthy nutrients instead of just excess calories.

Taking a Cue from Addiction Research

A sizable amount of research surrounding drug addiction is focused on the role of cravings in perpetuating the addictive cycle and how they can be reduced. Addiction literature is therefore a natural place to look for craving-reduction techniques. Strategies that help successfully combat the cravings that come with addiction may also be effective when it comes to food cravings. One such approach is the practice of mindfulness. In 2013, a group of current smokers who were hoping to quit their addiction were recruited to take part in a study in which they were either asked to simply look at pictures related to smoking, such as a lit cigarette, or "actively focus on their responses to the picture, including thoughts, feelings, memories, and bodily sensations, while maintaining a nonjudgmental attitude toward those responses." Participants in this condition were told to "notice and accept" how they responded to the images. The results of this study showed that compared to participants who looked passively at the images, the mindfulness group reported statistically lower levels of cravings after seeing the smoking cues. This demonstrates that although cravings might not be entirely avoidable, we can choose to intentionally respond to them, lessening their influence on how we feel, and thus potentially reducing the likelihood of giving into our impulses. Though this technique may take some getting used to, it could be helpful, the next time you experience a strong craving, to acknowledge and accept it—not give in to it or even fight it; just notice how you feel and accept it. This may help reduce its pull on you and allow you to more easily move past it.

Finally, while not necessarily craving-related, research into the topic of dietary habits during pregnancy has revealed a few calorie traps to look out for. In a recent study, some pregnant women reported replacing coffee with carbonated beverages or juices for that desired burst of energy. Likewise, some women chose these types of drinks when around friends and family who were drinking alcoholic beverages, either to avoid feeling left out or to calm their stomach if they felt nauseous. Regardless of any potential benefit, however, these drinks often contain large amounts of sugar. Thus these seemingly minor and even healthy-looking swaps may lead to excess calories and detrimental effects on your baby's developing body. To avoid this, try to brainstorm ahead of time to figure out which substitutions you might like that may serve the same purpose in these situations without adding extra sugar to your diet.

*　*　*

Now that we have covered the major hormones involved in stimulating appetite during pregnancy and some ways to handle food cravings, let's change gears a bit and discuss in more detail what you can do to keep your weight in check throughout pregnancy and once your baby is born.

CHAPTER 8

What You Can Do to Keep Your Weight Gain on Track during Pregnancy

Along with the many joys that accompany the anticipation of new life, expectant mothers may struggle with various questions surrounding weight gain. What can I do to prevent gaining too much weight and having a lot to lose once my baby is born? Is it safe to exercise during pregnancy? Concerns about weight gain can be anxiety provoking without the right information. In this chapter, I will expand on the recommended guidelines for weight gain during pregnancy that we first discussed in chapter 2, including how fast weight should be gained and suggestions for exercise during pregnancy, as well as other strategies to keep your weight on track during pregnancy.

In today's society, weight gain generally carries a negative connotation. However, how we conceptualize weight gain and the meaning we attach to it can transform the experience from one of dread to one of beauty. Weight gain during pregnancy is not ordinary weight gain. It is a necessity to create life, and we shouldn't forget that. It is necessary to support the proper development of your child's body and the storage of resources needed for lactation. When thought of in this way, the increasing numbers on the scale can be viewed as both necessary and even positive (within reason, of course). This last qualifier is an important one, which is why I start this chapter discussing in depth what "within reason" actually means: I've chosen to focus on weight gain during the second and third trimesters because although it is common to gain some weight in the first trimester (about 1 to 4½ pounds), most weight gain occurs during the later stages of pregnancy.

Weight Gain Guidelines for the Second Trimester

The second trimester is when your weight should start increasing at a much faster pace due to more rapid fetal growth, accumulating maternal stores, and an improved appetite. As detailed in chapter 2, gestational weight gain has been associated with a number of health outcomes for both mother and baby. In the second trimester specifically, studies show direct links between too little weight gain and having a "small for gestational age" baby, as well as too much gestational weight gain and having a "large for gestational age" baby. In addition, it appears that the timing of excessive weight gain during pregnancy can be important. Research shows that excess weight gain in the first half of pregnancy (up to 20 weeks) increases the amount of a baby's adipose tissue (fat) at birth, thus increasing the child's risk for obesity later in life. Therefore, gaining the recommended amount of weight and at an optimal rate is key for a healthy baby.

Remember, you are supposed to eat only an extra 340 calories each day (see page 76) during the second trimester, and that doesn't really amount to a lot of extra food each day. In terms of weight gain, as you may recall from chapter 2, how much weight you are advised to gain in total will vary depending on your prepregnancy BMI. You can see in the chart on the next page that the rate of weight gain over the second trimester may also vary depending on your prepregnancy BMI. Further, if you gained more than a few pounds in your first trimester, you may not gain at quite the same rate as you would if you didn't gain any weight during the first trimester. If your prepregnancy BMI was normal, you should plan to gain roughly 1 pound per week during the second trimester.

Weight Gain Guidelines for the Third Trimester

Unlike the second trimester, starting at around week 34 (gestation week 36), about half of the weight that you gain will be going directly to your baby. That is, for every pound that you gain, your baby will be gaining about half of it. In addition, more than half (about 70 percent) of all the energy that goes to your baby is going to its rapidly growing and developing brain.

So how much should you be gaining during the third trimester? Remember, during the third trimester you are supposed to eat only an extra 450 calories

what to eat when you're pregnant

Weight Gain throughout Pregnancy by BMI

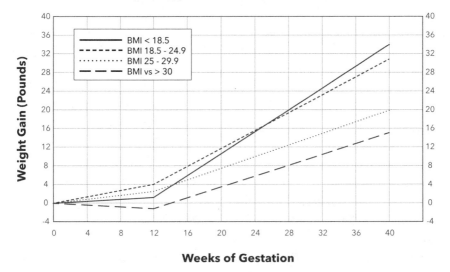

Source: Available at http://diabetes-pregnancy.ca/wp-content/uploads/2011/06/
Weight-Gain-Lbs.pdf. Accessed July 11, 2014.

(see page 105) each day (here's how little that can be: 1½ cups of whole milk and five Oreo cookies is around 450 calories). You can see from the chart above that the rate of weight gain over the third trimester may also vary depending on your prepregnancy BMI. If your prepregnancy BMI was normal, you should plan to gain roughly 1 pound per week during the third trimester (as you did in the second trimester, as well).

There are several studies that support the need to try and stay on track with your weight gain goals during the middle-to-latter part of your pregnancy. Excess weight gain during the second and third trimesters (regardless of BMI), as noted in chapter 2, has been associated with an increased chance of having a large for gestational age baby and a C-section delivery, among other risks. Both small and large for gestational age babies have an increased risk of being obese as children as well as later in life—another reason it is important to try and gain weight within the recommended guidelines for your BMI. It is also worth mentioning a recent study that found that increased gestational weight gain during the third trimester was associated with greater body weight of babies at 6 months old.

Weight Gain Chart

During one of your prenatal visits your doctor may have given you a gestational weight gain chart to track your pregnancy weight. In case you don't have a chart yet, one is included on page 145. This chart has four lines, one for each possible category of prepregnancy BMI (underweight, normal weight, overweight, and obese), and you need to pay attention to only the one that corresponds to your own prepregnancy BMI. You can see that at 12 weeks, the line rises steadily without plateaus until delivery, indicating the need for *steady* weight gain over this time frame. You can use this chart to track your weight gain as you go, marking your weight on the graph at each week and comparing it to the "recommendation line" appropriate for your BMI category.

Are you falling below or above the line? Don't stress out if you're a couple of pounds short or a couple of pounds over what the line recommends. If you gained 2 pounds in one week, you may gain none or less than 1 pound in the following week, and things will eventually even out. In addition, the Institute of Medicine expresses gestational weight gain recommendations as ranges instead of specific numbers. Gaining 5 pounds more or less at the end of pregnancy (the line for the normal BMI category ends at 30 pounds, but weight gain anywhere from 25 to 35 is considered optimal), as long as it falls within the recommended range, is not thought to contribute to negative outcomes. However, if you find that you're "off the chart" and it's only the beginning of the second trimester, or if the pounds appear to be piling on by the days instead of by the weeks, you should speak to your doctor; there may be an underlying issue causing rapid weight gain, such as fluid accumulation. Next, evaluate your dietary and exercise habits. Are you consuming a balanced diet? Or do you find yourself overindulging whenever a craving strikes? Are you getting enough physical activity? Drinking plenty of water? All of these factors can lead to a more rapid than recommended weight gain.

HOW MUCH WATER DO YOU NEED DURING PREGNANCY? ——

Although your fluid intake recommendations during pregnancy are not different from what is suggested when you are not pregnant (eight 8-ounce glasses per day, or 64 ounces), it is a good idea to try to meet this goal and to have your fluids largely be from water. Water can be your friend during pregnancy for several reasons. Drinking water can help minimize constipation, hemorrhoids, and bladder infections, and decrease swelling (oddly, the more water you drink, the less you retain). So drink up!

what to eat when you're pregnant

Preventing Excessive Weight Gain during Pregnancy

Over the past decade or so, an abundance of studies have emerged investigating whether behavioral lifestyle interventions can be helpful in reducing excessive weight gain during pregnancy, so we can really see *what works*. According to these studies, programs that promote healthy diets and increased physical activity are effective in reducing excess gestational weight gain. Interestingly, this effect appears to be even greater if expectant moms also monitor their weight or have an established maximum weight gain in mind. This shared focus on diet, physical activity, and weight seems to have a trifecta effect when it comes to limiting weight gain during pregnancy. So, consider joining a group that is focused on weight goals. Your ob-gyn will likely have some local group contact information (or may in fact run one herself).

THE CHECKS AND BALANCES OF YOUR WEIGHT ───────────

Let's say eating is like spending money and exercise is like saving it. If you check your bank account balance (aka body weight) at consistent intervals, you'll know if and when you've been spending more than you're saving, can reflect on how or why this has been happening, and can adjust your behavior instead of suddenly finding out you're nearing bankruptcy. This is why simple tools like the weight gain chart (see page 145) can be so helpful in preventing or reducing too much weight gain.

A few variables are linked with excessive gestational weight gain that we have little control over, such as age and whether or not it's your first pregnancy. However, in a study of more than a thousand expectant women, researchers noted a number of modifiable factors that predicted whether women would gain excessive weight during pregnancy. First, they found that greater caloric intake in general and greater consumption of fried food (think French fries) and dairy items (think ice cream) in particular were associated with excessive weight gain. What does this mean for you? Ice cream and fries once in a while as a treat are fine, but if these foods are dominating your diet, you need to make a change. Also, studies of people eating a vegetarian diet found it was protective against gaining too much weight. So, while I am not suggesting you go full vegetarian for this reason, you might consider going meatless one or two days each week. Studies also show that walking and engaging in other regular physical activity helped shield women from excessive gains. This underscores why it is so important to stay active during your pregnancy. Even walking counts!

Additional direction comes from a recent study showing that compared to standard health care, engaging in a behavioral program aimed at improving and monitoring both diet and physical activity levels of expecting moms helped reduce excessive gestational weight gain in women of normal weight. This intervention program consisted of a number of techniques (in addition to standard care), including setting goals to increase physical activity (30 minutes of walking most days) and to decrease consumption of high-fat foods, and following a carefully outlined diet plan based on the prescribed weight gain. Consistent with the trifecta effect mentioned earlier, expectant mothers in this study were also advised to monitor their weight and food intake and to exercise daily, using body weight scales, food records, and pedometers. In light of these positive results, it may be worth it to try some (or all!) of these methods to keep your weight in check during pregnancy.

A 2013 study conducted in Ireland suggests that certain types of food may also help prevent the pounds from piling on. This study compared pregnant women given standard maternity care to those who were given healthy dietary advice and encouraged to trade high glycemic index (GI) foods for those with a low GI. The glycemic index is a system of classifying carbohydrates based on how quickly they break down in your body and release glucose—the main building block for your baby's development—into your bloodstream. Examples of high-GI foods include white bread or rice; examples of low-GI foods include whole grain bread and apples. In this study, women in the dietary intervention group were significantly less likely to exceed the Institute of Medicine guidelines for gestational weight gain. Along with consuming fewer calories overall, these women tended to consume fewer high-calorie drinks, refined breakfast cereals, and white bread, and consumed more whole grain breads and cereals, protein, fiber, oily fish, and yogurt, with a higher intake of vitamin A and magnesium. And to make this shift in food patterns even better, the women gave positive feedback when asked about their feelings about the changes they made to their diet as part of the study. In fact, the majority of women said that they enjoyed making the changes and felt they had a wide variety of foods to eat and their diets provided enough energy.

SHOULD I FOLLOW A LOW-GI DIET WHILE PREGNANT? ———

While not all studies have found a difference in weight gain between dietary groups, there is some evidence—though it remains mixed—that expecting mothers who consume a low-GI diet may be less likely to deliver babies who are large for gestational age and have increased body fat compared to expecting mothers who consume a high-GI diet. Children born large for gestational age also tend to weigh more 2 years post delivery. On the opposite end of the spectrum, a low-GI diet may raise the risk of having a small for gestational age child—suggesting that moderation is key. It is possible that a low-GI diet might be especially beneficial for overweight or obese mothers-to-be, as they have an increased chance of delivering a large for gestational age child. Furthermore, some (but not all) research has shown that a diet consisting of low-GI foods can reduce the need to receive insulin in women with gestational diabetes.

Interventions shown to be effective in normal weight pregnant women do not always show the same effect in overweight or obese pregnant women. Fortunately, however, studies have begun to fill this gap, providing several insights into what is effective for women who fall into these weight categories. First, it turns out that just having an accurate assessment of your prepregnancy BMI may actually be helpful in avoiding excess weight gain while pregnant. A study published in 2008 found that women with an overweight or obese prepregnancy BMI who underestimated how much they weighed prior to pregnancy were more likely to gain excessive weight during pregnancy. Eighty percent of overweight and obese pregnant women avoided gaining excessive gestational weight when following another study's program, which encouraged them to consume approximately 2,000 calories per day, of which 40 to 50 percent were from carbohydrates (especially complex carbs and low-GI foods), 30 percent were from fat (especially monounsaturated fatty acids instead of saturated and trans fats), and 20 to 30 percent were from protein. In addition to this diet plan, the women were encouraged to walk three or four times per week, initially for 25 minutes and eventually for 40 minutes at a time, and were given a pedometer to track their steps. Also, obese women who enrolled in a program that offered motivational, informational, and supportive sessions each week, along with one or two aqua aerobic classes each week, gained less weight during pregnancy than obese women who received routine care, and these women had significantly lower BMIs at postnatal checkups at 10 to 12 weeks postpartum.

NEED HELP STAYING ON TRACK?

If you find that you aren't able to maintain your eating habits and weight gain goals, you might want to enlist the help of a nutritionist. Research has shown that pregnant women with obesity who attended ten one-hour sessions with a dietitian and were encouraged to eat according to dietary recommendations were better able to limit their weight gain compared to women who were not seeing a nutritionist. Therefore, regularly meeting with a dietitian throughout pregnancy, along with making the necessary adjustments to your diet, can be beneficial in protecting against too much weight gain.

In addition to considering health- and energy-related factors, psychological factors play a role in pregnancy weight gain. When obese women are encouraged to identify behaviors that they could change, discuss their personal barriers to change, and set reasonable goals, and are given positive affirmations in order to build confidence (along with lessons in how to read a food label), there is a decrease in both weight gain and anxiety levels of the expectant mothers.

So while it is important to focus on diet and exercise while pregnant, it may also be valuable to consider how these tools relate to you personally. Take some time to consider *how* you might benefit from changing, the barriers that may be keeping you from making these changes, and strategies for you to overcome those barriers. And though it may sound silly, support yourself during this journey! If you find you are struggling to make big changes in your diet or exercise habits, try to set small goals that you can accomplish for the next week, to build a sense of self-efficacy. And when you succeed, acknowledge your accomplishment! This can lay the groundwork for a positive feedback loop that will continue to reinforce healthy decisions going forward.

Is It Safe to Exercise during Pregnancy? You Bet!

Though most women want to prevent gaining too much weight during the course of their pregnancy, some may wonder whether exercise is a safe way to control their weight. To answer this question, a group of researchers in Spain assigned two hundred pregnant women to either an exercise or a control group, with the exercise group engaging in about one hour of physical activity three days per week. The results showed that women in the exercise group were less likely to gain excessive weight, and further, maternal and neonatal health outcomes did not differ between the two groups, indicating that this level of moderate exercise did not put the women or babies at a higher risk for complications. In fact, the American Congress of Obstetricians and Gynecologists issued a statement, which was reaffirmed in 2009, indicating that pregnant women without medical or obstetric complications can also follow the Centers for Disease Control and American College of Sports Medicine guidelines for exercise for nonpregnant individuals: at least 30 minutes of moderate exercise each day (on most or all days of the week). Several studies have now confirmed these findings: Physical activity during pregnancy is safe and is also effective in reducing gestational weight gain.

Now that doesn't mean you should start training for a marathon! "Physical activity" doesn't mean that your workouts have to be super intense to be effective. In one study, pregnant women with normal BMIs who were asked to walk three or four times a week (for 15 to 30 minutes, not including warm-up or cool-down time) at either a low or moderate intensity (based on heart rate) gained significantly less weight during pregnancy than women who were not physically active. In fact, excessive weight gain was prevented in 70 percent and 77 percent of mothers-to-be in the low and moderate-intensity groups, respectively. As an added bonus, these women were less apt to retain as much weight after delivery than those who were not enrolled in the exercise program.

Further evidence of the benefits conferred by exercise during pregnancy comes from a study that found that light- to moderate-intensity physical activity (aerobic and resistance exercises three times a week for 50 to 55 minutes each) helped normal weight pregnant women gain less weight than a control group. In fact, women in the exercise group were 40 percent less likely to exceed the Institute of Medicine guidelines during pregnancy! Moreover, exercise may have a positive impact on pregnancy symptoms; another study in obese pregnant women found that women who exercised (defined as burning more than 900 calories through exercise each week) were less likely to experience nausea and lower back pain.

BUMP-FRIENDLY EXERCISE IDEAS

Here are some ideas for exercises you can do during your pregnancy and beyond. Sometimes doing the same old exercise can get boring, so if that happens to you, try one of these instead!

Gentle or prenatal yoga. Take a class, pop in a DVD, or cue up YouTube. If you take a class, be sure to let the instructor know you are expecting. He or she may suggest some alternative poses.

Walking. Take Fido outside in the fresh air. A brisk walk can be invigorating and is beneficial to your health. If you need some motivation, enlist a neighbor or a friend to start a ritual of taking an evening walk.

Swimming. Swimming is easy on your joints, and in the summer months it can give you welcome relief from the heat. It works arm and leg muscles at the same time and is a great cardiovascular workout. Plus, it feels nice to float around weightless in a pool, especially when you start feeling those added pounds from your pregnancy.

Not into exercising? Don't worry; you can burn calories in more creative (and productive) ways. Cleaning the house can burn up to 80 calories in 20 minutes. So much the better if the "nesting syndrome" hits and you feel the need to have everything in your house spic-and-span before the little one arrives.

Dance! Everyone loves to dance, and it can be great exercise, too. Twenty minutes of dancing (depending on the type) can burn up to 100 calories.

Join Baby Boot Camp (www.BabyBootCamp.com). There are several groups of moms out there who get together to work out, with their strollers! The exercises are fun and purposefully designed to be entertaining for little ones who may be tagging along. Not only is this a fun and stress-free way to work out, but it is also a great way to meet other new moms with children the same age. My favorite class is Strolloga (that is yoga with a stroller). If you don't have any children yet, you can still participate. Bring your empty stroller and join in the fun. Plus, you can have an exciting activity to participate in together after the new baby arrives!

*   *   *

In this chapter I discussed the guidelines regarding how much weight to gain over your pregnancy and offered some ways in which you can keep your weight in check during this time. In the next chapter, I will talk about what you can do to speed up losing your "baby weight" once the little one has arrived.

CHAPTER 9

Losing Your Baby Weight and Maintaining a Healthy Diet beyond the Bump

Now that your baby is out of your belly and in your arms, you may be overwhelmed with all the changes that are happening in your life. Understandably so: a new baby in the house, maybe breastfeeding, an altered sleep schedule (which is a major understatement), maternity leave (or planning to return to work), never-ending diaper changes, and other chores all result in a serious deviation from what was considered "the norm" just weeks, or even days, before. You may also be starting to wonder when all those pounds that you gained during pregnancy are going to melt away. With all of your new responsibilities in life, the last thing you want to deal with is losing weight.

In this chapter, I discuss what you should expect regarding postpartum weight loss, how to maintain a healthy eating pattern amid the changes that accompany your new bundle of joy, and tips for staying energized, well nourished, and happy in the years to come.

The Truth about Post-Pregnancy Weight Loss

Are you ready for this? Because I'm going to tell you the cold, hard truth. You will still look pregnant when you leave the hospital. Not *as* pregnant as when you checked in, but pregnant nonetheless. Remember those photos of Giselle Bündchen in a bikini that I mentioned in chapter 1, where she looked no different from before getting pregnant? Well, as it turns out, that same miraculous weight loss doesn't appear to happen to us mere mortals. I am embarrassed to admit this, but when I had my daughter, I foolishly assumed (read: dreamed) that like Giselle, I would go home from the hospital wearing not maternity clothes, but a pair of my old fat jeans (and I just knew I'd be back into my regular jeans in no time). Boy, was I ever wrong! I had to send my husband home to get some clothes that actually fit me before I could leave the maternity ward.

In the days following delivery, you will still have a bump, and even though it won't be nearly as big as it was before, it will take its time in saying goodbye. That's okay! It is perfectly natural and normal, so don't spend time stressing about it. You actually shouldn't attempt to lose weight until (1) a proper breastfeeding pattern is established (if you will be nursing), (2) your uterus has shrunk back to its normal size, and (3) your doctor gives you the okay to start exercising. After a vaginal delivery, you can usually start engaging in mild to moderate exercise as soon as you feel up for it (this could be within days after delivery). If you have a Cesarean, it will take a bit longer before you can resume physical activity, as your abdominal muscles and scar need to heal properly. Your doctor will determine when you can get back to your regular exercise routine, but most women are able to start moderate exercise 6 to 8 weeks post-Cesarean. Regardless, you will need some time to get yourself used to your new role as a mom, so don't rush into worrying about losing weight.

As you may remember from previous chapters, gaining the recommended amount of weight during pregnancy means a faster bouncing back to your pre-pregnancy body and weight. However, regardless of how much weight you gained while expecting, you will lose approximately 12 pounds with the birth of your baby (I lost 11), and a few more in the several days or weeks following delivery due to the normal loss of fluids that you accumulated during pregnancy.

Where Was That Weight From?
Weight Loss in the First Week or Two after Delivery

Baby	6 to 8 pounds (although can vary)
Placenta	1 to 2 pounds
Amniotic fluid	2 to 3 pounds
Blood	Less than a pound
Water	3 to 4 pounds in the first week (can vary depending on how much water you retained, may be lost in the first few days or a couple of weeks)

TOTAL: 12 to 18 pounds, about 12 of which are lost during delivery

what to eat when you're pregnant

Recall the gestational weight gain breakdown in chapter 2 (see page 21): the pounds you gained during pregnancy went to a variety of places in your body, and many of these will not automatically drop off at birth or in the several days after. These include your enlarged breasts and uterus, increased blood volume, and fat stores. Your uterus will start to shrink right after giving birth and will eventually decrease to its normal size after 6 to 8 weeks postpartum. The blood volume will also decrease, as you no longer need an increased blood supply to nourish the baby growing inside of you. However, the nutrient stores (a much nicer term than "fat") that you have accumulated will take their time before departing. Remember: you didn't gain all the weight in one day, so you shouldn't expect it to go away overnight. I have heard people use the expression "9 months on and 9 months off." That is a fair and realistic goal. In addition, other factors, like diet, exercise, and whether or not you breastfed, will influence the rate of your weight loss.

Statistics about Postpartum Weight Loss

According to the Pregnancy Nutrition Surveillance System, which collected data on about forty-nine thousand women in the United States between 2004 and 2006, the average postpartum weight retention, or the weight retained by women at around 6 months postpartum, was 11.8 pounds. About half of women retained more than 10 pounds, and one-quarter retained more than 20 pounds. Weight retention varied by race, with African American women retaining more weight than white or Hispanic women, regardless of their pre-pregnancy BMI or gestational weight gain. Among women who gained more than the Institute of Medicine recommendations, the average postpartum weight retention was 15 to 20 pounds. At later points after delivery, another study of American women showed that at 11 to 14 months post-pregnancy only a quarter of women retained more than 10 pounds, although 12 percent of all women still retained more than 20 pounds. On the other side of the equator, a survey of Brazilian women (18 to 45 years old) showed that the mean weight retention 9 months post-pregnancy was only about 6.8 pounds. Women over 30 tended to retain more weight than younger women, and breastfeeding was associated with weight loss in women of all ages but not in those who were obese prior to becoming pregnant.

What can we make of all these statistics, and how can they help predict your post-pregnancy weight loss? First of all, if you gain weight within the recommended range during pregnancy, your odds of losing it after delivery are already increased. Additionally, if you are breastfeeding, your pounds are likely to disappear faster. Third, if you are African American, you may lose weight more slowly than mothers who are Caucasian or Hispanic. Again, this statistic does not mean this will be the case; it just makes it more likely, and having this awareness may help you stay motivated and reduce your likelihood of slower weight loss. Bottom line? Be patient and don't stress. With healthy eating skills and exercise routines, and using the tips to avoid falling into craving traps mentioned in chapter 7 (which you can carry with you beyond delivery), you will bounce back to your previous body and weight over time.

Strategies for Losing the Bump after Your Baby Is Born

Here are several ideas for things you can do to help speed the process of losing your baby weight. Remember, slow and steady wins the race.

Gain the Right Amount of Weight during Pregnancy

One of the easiest ways to up your odds of returning to your original weight after your baby is born is, of course, to not gain too much during pregnancy. In fact, one study found weight gain during pregnancy to be the strongest predictor of postpartum weight retention a year after delivery. This is why implementing healthy changes like eating a nutritious diet and engaging in regular, moderate exercise during pregnancy actually serve double duty: they tend to prevent gaining too much weight and thus reduce the amount of weight you need to lose once your baby is born. These changes can also establish a set of habits so that after your baby is born you don't have to initiate a whole new routine. This may be why a 2014 study of women with obesity who followed a walking program throughout their pregnancy showed less weight retention at 6 months postpartum compared to a control group.

Get Physical

Relatedly, and somewhat unsurprisingly, exercise is often associated with less postpartum weight retention. While this seems like a no-brainer, getting in enough time for physical activity once your baby is born may be tough. Between being up repeatedly in the middle of the night, possibly resuming some of your responsibilities at work, and a potentially new challenge of finding reliable childcare, just scheduling a workout can seem exhausting. Not to fear! There are a number of ways to overcome these obstacles so you can get back into shape. Taking your baby on a walk or jog using a stroller, for instance, can be a great way to get moving without having to hire a babysitter. In fact, just walking 30 or more minutes per day (as well as watching less than 2 hours of television per day) is associated with less weight retention. Added benefits: your little one may find the ride relaxing (and may take a nap!), you are both out in the fresh air, and you are setting a good example from day one that exercise is important.

Another way to get some exercise with your baby nearby is to watch (and participate in) a fitness DVD or an online workout. If you find it difficult to carve out enough time for the gym or an exercise class between home and work responsibilities, take a few minutes each week to schedule your workouts ahead of time, then hold yourself to them. The bottom line is that if it is important to you, it is important. If you need to call on your partner or friends and family to take over while you do something beneficial for your health, do it! If you needed more convincing, research has found associations between exercise at 6 months after delivery and better psychosocial well-being, including greater satisfaction with motherhood, the quality of your relationship with your partner, and your life circumstances more generally.

Breastfeed

Around 75 percent of new mothers in the United States breastfeed, a choice that is strongly supported by the American Congress of Obstetrics and Gynecologists. While research on the link between breastfeeding and postpartum weight retention remains mixed, a number of studies suggest that this practice may be helpful in shedding pregnancy pounds. In fact, it has been suggested that if done as recommended, breastfeeding may be able to eliminate postpartum weight retention within just 6 months in women who gain a reasonable amount (approximately 26 pounds) while pregnant. It should be noted, however, that the weight loss effect of breastfeeding appears to be less pronounced among women who are obese prepregnancy.

Eat Healthfully

Although your life after giving birth may be a bit hectic, maintaining healthy eating patterns is crucial for shedding those extra pounds. Women who began snacking more between meals (meaning three or more snacks a day) after pregnancy have been shown to retain greater weight postpartum; the same is true for women who began skipping meals after giving birth. In addition to the importance of *how* you eat, studies show that *what* you eat can influence weight loss after pregnancy, with research finding less weight retention among women who consume fewer trans fats. Likewise, a recent study found greater losses of postpartum weight among women who consumed less junk food—like fast food and soda—and ate more nutritious foods, like fruits, vegetables, and milk. So what can you do to eat healthy? Read on!

How to Maintain a Healthy Eating Pattern Post-Pregnancy

While the focus has been on weight, note that the ultimate goal is to be healthy. Taking care of your little one is most likely consuming the majority of your time, so maintaining a healthy diet may seem daunting, at best. Fortunately, you learned a great deal about eating well during your pregnancy, so you don't need to learn a ton of new information now that your baby is born. The key is to maintain the same healthy eating habits that you have been adhering to throughout your pregnancy. The main change now is the lack of time, making good time-management skills key. However, the good news is that, despite the common belief, eating healthy and having limited time aren't incompatible! To stay well nourished and energized in the weeks following your baby's birth, when things may seem crazy around the house, consider the following tips.

Choose Rapid Recipes

In the first few days or weeks after giving birth, you may not have the time, energy, or willingness to spend much time in the kitchen. However, that doesn't mean that the only other options are fast food or other suboptimal, convenience foods. Fortunately, wholesome meals do not always need hours of preparation! Recall that many of the recipes in this book can be prepared in thirty minutes or less.

To save time, opt for foods that can be eaten raw, such as fresh vegetables or a quick salad. Also, frozen and canned foods can be a great option, as they usually need only to be heated up or cooked for a short time after thawing. However, pay attention to the ingredients that may have been added to these convenience foods, such as sodium (canned foods are notorious for this), and choose those that have little if any additives. Finally, presoak your grains and legumes before cooking them—this will dramatically decrease cooking time.

And if you do spend a little while in the kitchen one day, try to make enough to last for a couple of days (requiring only reheating), which will save you time in the next day or two.

Make Quick and Wholesome Breakfasts

It is tempting to think we can save some calories by skipping breakfast. This isn't true. Skipping breakfast leads to increased hunger later on, which can lead to poor food choices. Also, studies show that breakfast skippers are not more likely to lose weight; in fact, skipping breakfast can lead to weight gain.

An essential meal of the day, breakfast can be highly nutritious while also being quick and easy to prepare. Quick and easy are critical elements, especially when your alarm clock is most likely your hungry baby! Enriched, low-sugar breakfast cereals with skim milk and fresh fruit, fruit and vegetable smoothies with low-fat yogurt, and eggs (any style) with whole grain toast are all excellent choices that only take about 5 minutes to make and are simple enough to prepare even with a baby strapped close in a sling or pack (or later, on your hip). Even though your sleeping patterns (and your general schedule) may be less than ideal at this time, try to eat breakfast around the same time each day to keep energized and help you stick to a breakfast-eating pattern, boosting your metabolism from the beginning of the day. In addition, eating breakfast has been linked to weight loss and weight loss maintenance, as well as improved nutrient intake, so try your best to eat a nutrient-dense breakfast each day to help you shed the baby weight more easily.

KEEP HEALTHY SNACKS AT HOME,
IN YOUR BAG, AND IN THE DIAPER BAG ————————————————

Fresh fruit, vegetables, yogurt, whole grain (and low-sugar) granola and energy bars, and smoothies all make healthy snacks. As men-tioned in chapter 7, it can be especially helpful to keep a few of these handy at all times. Your appetite may be really powerful these days, especially if you are breastfeeding, so having healthy snacks within reach will keep you from turning to the not-so-healthy, quick-fix options. And because your body may pine for different things at different times, try to stock up on a variety of your favorite healthy foods so you have a nice selection.

Stay Hydrated

Essential in every stage of life, drinking plenty of water and keeping yourself hydrated is especially important in the postpartum period. Drinking water requires little time but may take a little bit of planning, considering all the things you now have to juggle. Be sure to always have a glass or bottle of water around wherever you are. If you are breastfeeding, you may want to keep a glass of water nearby and sip on it as you're feeding your baby. You need a lot of fluids when you breastfeed, as the majority of your milk is composed of water. Try not to wait until you actually feel the sensation of thirst (at that point, your body is already about 2 percent dehydrated), and drink frequently throughout the day. Not only will this keep you properly hydrated, but it will also ensure that you feel good (dehydration can cause headaches, cramps, constipation, and other things that you don't want to deal with at this time).

Eat during the Day

With all the waking, singing, cradling, and feeding you are now doing in the wee hours of night, you may find yourself also snacking then. Midnight snacking can contribute to an excess of calories and thus potentially prolong the amount of time needed to shed those remaining pounds. In addition, eating when you get up during the night and then going back to bed can prevent you from getting good, quality sleep. It may sound like that's impossible in the first place, but eating shortly before sleeping means your body is working on digesting, which prevents your brain from entering deep sleep, which is the kind of sleep that recharges you and makes you feel well rested in the morning.

Utilize Your Support System

Your partner, parents, other kids, siblings, and other family or friends can be invaluable in many different ways at this time, and helping you to eat healthy is one of them. Do not be shy to ask for help if you need it! Grocery shopping may seem like mission impossible in the first few days or weeks after delivery (especially after a Cesarean), so don't hesitate to ask a family member or

what to eat when you're pregnant

friend to pick up your groceries for you. In addition, you can reach out for some cooking assistance, especially if you have a friend or family member who loves to do it (and is good at it!).

Healthy Eating beyond the Postpartum Period

Your healthy eating habits should not end when your baby is 3, 6, or even 12 months old; you can use your knowledge of nutrition to continue to eat healthily going forward. The principles of optimal nutrition after pregnancy and breastfeeding are not radically different from what they were during those periods; if anything, they are more relaxed, as certain foods and drinks that were forbidden when you were pregnant (such as moderate intake of alcohol or chicken salad from a deli) are perfectly compatible with a healthy, balanced diet. In addition, while your diet should still be nutrient-dense and contain all the vitamins, minerals, and nutrients that your body needs, the requirements for their intake are not as rigorous, since suboptimal intake won't have the same consequences as it might have had during pregnancy.

Yet most of us—mothers included—consume much less of what we should and too much of what we shouldn't. Our intakes of whole grains, vegetables, fruits, dairy, seafood, and healthy oils are all below the recommended levels. Similarly, the intakes of fiber and other nutrients that are critical for good health, including potassium, vitamin D, and calcium, are also below the recommended daily levels. On the other hand, foods and nutrients that should be avoided or consumed in moderation—like refined grains, sodium, and saturated fatty acids—are often consumed more often than recommended. What can you do to ensure that your dietary intake levels fall on or close to your goal? The rest of this chapter will focus on exactly that, offering you specific tips on how to maintain a healthy dietary pattern over the long term.

How Do Typical American Diets Compare to Recommended Intake Levels or Limits?

Usual intake as a percentage of goal or limit

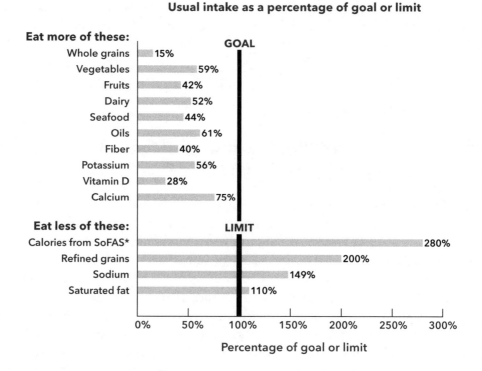

Percentage of goal or limit

SoFAS = solid fats and added sugars.

Note: Bars show average intakes for all individuals (ages 1 or 2 years or older, depending on the data source) as a percentage of the recommended intake level or limit. Recommended intakes for food groups and limits for refined grains and solid fats and added sugars are based on amounts in the USDA 2,000-calorie food pattern. Recommended intakes for fiber, potassium, vitamin D, and calcium are based on the highest adequate intake or recommended daily allowance for ages 14 to 70 years. Limits for sodium are based on the upper limit and for saturated fat on 10% of calories. The protein foods group is not shown here because, on average, intake is close to recommended levels.

Source: U.S. Department of Agriculture and U.S. Department of Health and Human Services. Dietary Guidelines for Americans, 2010 (7th ed.) (Washington, DC: U.S. Government Printing Office, December 2010).

what to eat when you're pregnant

Understanding Food Labels

In order to eat healthily, it is important to know exactly what all the foods and drinks you consume actually contain. After reading Part II of this book, you may know a good deal about the nutrients contained in different foods, especially whole foods. However, not all foods are whole, unprocessed foods. This section is designed to help you become acquainted with the different aspects of the nutrition facts label that is printed on the package of every processed food.

Every nutrition facts label provides information about the contents of exactly *one serving* of that food, which is defined in the first line, right below the title "Nutrition Facts." This is important to keep in mind when reading a nutrition label, because you may be consuming more than what the manufacturer has determined to be one serving. On some beverages, for instance, the nutrition label may also indicate that there are 1.5 or 2 servings per bottle or container. Therefore, if you plan to drink the entire bottle, you must multiply the values listed on the label by 1.5 or 2 to see how much you are *really* consuming.

The second piece of information listed on a nutrition label is the number of calories per serving, located on the left-hand side. On the right side of this row, it shows how many of these calories come from fat. You may want to moderate your intake of foods with the majority of their calories coming from fats to maintain a healthy daily fat intake, which should be 20 to 35 percent of all your calories.

Next, the label provides a breakdown of the nutrients in the food, indicated as both the actual amount of a nutrient present in one serving (on the left side) and a percentage of the daily recommended intake (Percent Daily Value) of that nutrient (on the right side).

Always pay attention to the amount of saturated and trans fat contained in the foods you eat. You should limit your intake of saturated fats to less than 10 percent of all your calories, which in a 2,000 calories/day diet translates to less than 200 calories from saturated fats, or less than 22 g of saturated fat. And you should try to completely avoid trans fats, since they don't confer any health benefits. On the contrary, they can only damage your health by increasing your risk for cancer and other chronic illnesses. Thankfully, the manufacturers of most processed food products in the United States have now eliminated or are in the process of eliminating trans fats.

Be mindful of the cholesterol and sodium content, as you want to limit your intake of both to maintain good health (excess cholesterol intake contributes to cardiovascular disease, and excess sodium leads to high blood pressure, or hypertension).

The next piece of information is the carbohydrate content. This includes total carbohydrate, dietary fiber, and sugar content per serving. It is a good idea to choose foods with more fiber and less sugars to help you achieve the recommended daily intake of fiber and limit the calories from added sugars, which, if consumed in excess, may lead to weight gain.

Nutrition Facts

Serving Size 1 Bar (40g)

Check Calories

Amount Per Serving

Calories 170	Calories from Fat 60

	% Daily Value*
Total Fat 7g	**11**%
Saturated Fat 3g	**15**%
Trans Fat 0g	
Cholesterol 0mg	**0**%
Sodium 160mg	**7**%
Total Carbohydrate 24g	**8**%
Dietary Fiber 3g	**12**%
Sugars 10g	
Protein 5g	

Limit These Nutrients

Get Enough of These Nutrients

Vitamin A 2%	•	Vitamin C 2%
Calcium 20%	•	Iron 8%

*Percent Daily Values are based on a 2,000-calorie diet. Your daily values may be higher or lower depending on your calorie needs:

	Calories:	2,000	2,500
Total Fat	Less than	65g	80g
Sat Fat	Less than	20g	25g
Cholesterol	Less than	300mg	300mg
Sodium	Less than	2,400mg	2,400mg
Total Carbohydrate		300g	375g
Dietary Fiber		25g	30g

Calories per gram:
Fat 9 • Carbohydrate 4 • Protein 4

Ingredients: Granola Bar (Brown Rice Syrup, Granola [rolled oats, honey, canola oil], Dry Roasted Peanuts, Soy Crisps [soy protein isolate, rice flour, malt extract, calcium carbonate], Crisp Brown Rice [organic brown rice flour, evaporated cane juice, molasses, rice bran extract, sea salt], Glycerine, Peanut Butter [ground dry roasted peanuts], Inulin, Whey Protein Isolate, Gold Flax Seeds, Quinoa Flakes, Calcium Carbonate, Salt, Natural Flavors, Water, Soy Lecithin [an emulsifier]), Dark Compound Coating (evaporated cane juice, palm kernel oil, cocoa [processed with alkali], palm oil, soy lecithin [an emulsifier]).

Source: U.S. Department of Agriculture and U.S. Department of Health and Human Services. Dietary Guidelines for Americans, 2010 (7th ed.) (Washington, DC: U.S. Government Printing Office, December 2010).

what to eat when you're pregnant

The last macronutrient listed on the label is protein. According to the National Research Council, women between the ages of 19 and 70 should consume approximately 46 g of protein per day, but that amount can vary based on activity levels (less is needed if you are active, more if you are very active). In general, protein intake in adult women should be 10 to 35 percent of all calories.

Listed next are the four vitamins and minerals required to be reported on each food package: vitamins A and C, calcium, and iron. These are expressed as percentages of the daily recommended intake. However, it is important to keep in mind that all values in a nutrition facts label are based on a diet consisting of 2,000 calories per day (the amount of calories that an *average* person needs each day). If your daily energy goal is higher or lower than 2,000 calories, your needs for the nutrients will also differ accordingly. With that said, this label is still a useful guide to help you better understand the nutrient density of that food. Remember, nutrient-dense foods are those that deliver the most beneficial nutrients with relatively few calories (for example, 1 cup of kale is more nutrient-dense than a cupcake). Also, toward the bottom of the label there is a small table comparing the Percent Daily Values of a 2,000 calories per day and a 2,500 calories per day diet, indicating the different amounts for some nutrients. Note that the Percent Daily Values for cholesterol and sodium do not vary with different caloric intakes, as 300 mg of cholesterol and 2,400 mg of sodium are the upper limits of these daily recommended amounts (although less sodium should be consumed by those with certain conditions such as high blood pressure).

The last part of the label indicates the number of calories per gram of each macronutrient: carbohydrate and protein each have 4 calories per gram, while fat has 9 calories per gram.

HOW MANY CALORIES ARE IN A GRAM OF ALCOHOL? ———

Alcohol does not fall into any of the three macronutrient (protein, carbohydrate, and fat) calorie categories; it comes at an "energy price" of 7 calories per gram. A glass of wine can contain between 95 calories (6 ounces of light white wine) and 290 calories (3 ounces of dessert wine), a glass of beer can contain between 95 calories (12 ounces of light beer) and 360 calories (12 ounces of Imperial IPA), and a single shot of hard liquor (1.5 ounces) can contain about 100 calories (but more if mixed with juice or soda such as in a cocktail).

This may seem like a lot to remember. It is. It is also one of the main reasons why you are better off doing your best to avoid processed foods.

However, we both know that completely avoiding them is not realistic for most people. While you don't have to read the list of ingredients included at the bottom of a nutrition label each time you buy the same food (although ingredients do change from time to time in the same food product, often without an indication, especially when it comes to food additives or an increase in the sugar or fat content), it is a good habit when choosing between products to determine which is the healthiest option. Some nutritionists say that you should avoid foods that have more than five ingredients. While this can be very true for certain foods that contain additives, emulsifiers, food dyes, preservatives, thickening agents, flavor enhancers, or added sugars and fats, more does not necessarily mean worse when it comes to less-processed or whole foods, such as trail mix (some contain ten or more ingredients, all of which are perfectly healthy). So when examining a list of ingredients, look for words that aren't familiar or that make you wonder, *Why does this need to be in here?* Unfortunately, food manufacturers are often quite clever when it comes to hiding the bad stuff with terms that either may be unfamiliar to the average consumer or may sound healthy, which brings me to my next point . . .

Examples of Added Sugars That Can Be Listed as an Ingredient on a Food Label

Anhydrous dextrose	Lactose
Brown sugar	Malt syrup
Confectioner's (powdered) sugar	Maltose
Corn syrup	Molasses
Corn syrup solids	Nectars (e.g., peach nectar, pear nectar)
Dextrin	Pancake syrup
Fructose	Raw sugar
High-fructose corn syrup	Sucrose
Honey	Sugar
Invert sugar	White granulated sugar

Note: Other added sugars may be listed as an ingredient but are not recognized by the FDA as an ingredient name. These include cane juice, evaporated corn sweetener, fruit juice concentrate, crystal dextrose, glucose, liquid fructose, sugar cane juice, and fruit nectar.

Source: U.S. Department of Agriculture and U.S. Department of Health and Human Services. Dietary Guidelines for Americans, 2010 (7th ed.) (Washington, DC: U.S. Government Printing Office, December 2010).

Examples of Solid Fats That Can Be Listed as an Ingredient on a Food Label

Beef fat (tallow, suet)	Palm kernel oil
Butter	Palm oil
Chicken fat	Partially hydrogenated oils
Coconut oil	Pork fat (lard)
Cream	Shortening
Hydrogenated oils	Stick margarine

Note: The oils listed here are high in saturated fat, and partially hydrogenated oils contain trans fats; therefore, for nutritional purposes, these oils are considered solid fats.

Source: U.S. Department of Agriculture and U.S. Department of Health and Human Services. Dietary Guidelines for Americans, 2010 (7th ed.) (Washington, DC: U.S. Government Printing Office, December 2010).

Know Your Enemies

Food manufacturers use all sorts of lingo to disguise ingredients they know you know are not great for you. If a food contains sugar, for example, the label won't always list the word *sugar* as an ingredient. There are a plethora of other words that can be put on the label instead, and while those ingredients might have been made in different ways, essentially they are all considered as sugar on the label. Take a look at the table on the facing page, which lists some examples of names for added sugars that you may find in the ingredients list of a food label. Brown sugar may sound like a healthier alternative to white granulated sugar, but its effect on your body is basically the same, and it has the same nutritional value (or lack thereof) as regular white table sugar. Similarly, solid fats can be listed under a variety of names, which you can see in the table above. While *coconut oil* sounds much healthier than *pork fat,* they are both saturated fats that have similar effects on your health. When it comes to ingredients like sugars and fats, which we should consume in limited amounts, moderation is key. While the occasional bite won't kill you, try your best to avoid foods with added sugars, saturated fats, large amounts of sodium, and ingredients you can't pronounce.

Know Your Friends

Like added sugars and solid fats, healthy foods can sometimes be slightly hidden, yet unintentionally so. As you probably know by now, whole grains are healthy and should be consumed on a daily basis to provide you with the many nutrients they contain. However, you may not always spot them on a food label (although most foods will now boast of containing whole grains on the front of the package). Rolled oats, bulgur, millet, and popcorn (yup!) are all whole grains yet don't include the word "whole" in their names, making it less obvious. Take a look at the table below to see what other grains are whole grains and look for them when you read the ingredient list on a food package.

Examples of Whole Grains That Can Be Listed as an Ingredient on a Food Label

Brown rice	Whole grain barley
Buckwheat	Whole grain corn
Bulgur (cracked wheat)	Whole grain sorghum
Millet	Whole grain triticale
Oatmeal	Whole oats/oatmeal
Popcorn	Whole rye
Quinoa	Whole wheat
Rolled oats	Wild rice

Source: U.S. Department of Agriculture and U.S. Department of Health and Human Services. Dietary Guidelines for Americans, 2010 (7th ed.) (Washington, DC: U.S. Government Printing Office, December 2010).

Track Your Calorie Balance

Maintaining your weight means maintaining a calorie balance; that is, a balance between the calories you consume via foods and beverages and the calories you expend through physical activity and your body's metabolic processes. There's no need to count every calorie you eat, but if the number on your scale starts creeping upward (or if you're not at an ideal weight yet and are trying to reach it), you may want to track what you eat and how much energy you take in for a few days to get an idea of what areas you can target for improvement. To make this easier, there are now a variety of smartphone applications to choose from that will help you track your calorie and nutrient intake. These apps make entering information fast and easy, as you can search for the foods you eat by brand and select the exact amounts you've eaten. In addition, apps like these can help you see how what you're eating compares to your target calorie count as well as the recommended amounts of nutrients that you need. You can also use these apps to enter your weight, the amount of exercise you do, and other factors that can be helpful in supporting a healthy lifestyle.

Aim for Optimal Nutrient Proportions and Dietary Variety

You should aim to consume the recommended proportions of all three macro-nutrients, which for adults age 19 and older means that 45 to 65 percent of all daily calories should come from carbohydrates, 10 to 35 percent from protein, and 20 to 35 percent from fat. In addition, you should aim for variety in your diet instead of eating the same foods day after day. Consuming many different foods will not only help you increase the chances of getting all the nutrients you need but also reduce the risk of consuming too much of what your body does not need, such as mercury in fish.

Make the Most of Each Bite

Making the most of what you eat means getting the most nutrients per calorie, or the biggest bang for your buck. To do this, try to choose foods that are unprocessed or minimally processed, don't contain things you can't identify or pronounce, and contain little (if any) saturated and trans fats and added sugars while still offering you the flavor, texture, aroma, and other qualities that make food enjoyable. It is important to identify foods that meet all of these criteria, because more often than not flavor preference is the driving factor behind food selection (though price also plays a major role). Figuring out which foods offer all of these properties will help you maintain a healthy eating pattern in the long run.

Trick Yourself into Eating Well

Don't fancy all those raw leafy greens? While different preparation techniques can enhance the strong flavor of a food like collard greens, a quick and easy way to get everything that these nutrient-dense foods have to offer is to blend them into a smoothie. Adding fruits like bananas, strawberries, and pineapples will overpower the flavor of just about any leafy greens, yet still provide you with all the nutrients they contain. Try the smoothie recipes on page 95, or create your own. It's both easy and fun, since you can create an almost infinite spectrum of flavors (and textures), depending on the ingredients you include and the proportions you blend them in.

Don't Stress about Your Weight

This can be easier said than done, especially if you have a crying baby on your hands, a pile of laundry to fold, and a conference call for work in 2 minutes! But remember that stress is closely related to appetite. High stress levels can lead to an increased consumption of highly palatable foods, like foods high in sugar, fat, or both. Some researchers explain that repeated levels of high stress actually alter the way in which stress and appetite/energy are regulated in our brains, leading to stress-induced desire for and overeating of highly palatable foods, which in turn increases the risk of becoming overweight or obese. Try to avoid turning to food when you are stressed by using some of the techniques suggested in chapter 7.

It's the Big Picture That Matters

While all the little things—like what snacks you eat in the afternoon on any given day—certainly count, it's the overall pattern that matters most. The foods you regularly choose, the average amount of nutrients you get in the span of two or three days, the amount and frequency of alcoholic beverages you drink, the volume of water you drink, and the amount of fiber you consume with your food all make up your regular dietary pattern. If your *overall* dietary pattern is healthy, then a small piece of cake, a bowl of ice cream, or a candy bar every once in a while won't make much difference and won't lead to weight gain or obesity. That said, dessert and junk foods should remain occasional treats and not regularly eaten items.

* * *

In closing, it really *is* the big things that matter, and this extends well beyond your diet. Having a baby is one of those big things—the one that matters the most. I hope the information, tips, and recipes in this book have helped you think differently about food and view it as a way to help our little ones get the best start from the very beginning.

Appendix A:
Food Safety and Foods to
Avoid during Pregnancy

While the focus of this book is mainly on the positive changes you can make to your diet to improve the overall health and well-being of your growing baby, it is also important to discuss some of the key food safety issues. Pregnancy affects your immune system, increasing your and your baby's susceptibility to different bacteria, viruses, and parasites that may cause foodborne illnesses. So it's that much more important to focus on safe food handling, preparation, and consumption when you're pregnant. To decrease your risk of infection and prevent any potential harm to your baby, there are a few foods that you should avoid. Some of this may sound familiar, as it was mentioned in Part II when these food groups were discussed. However, when it comes to the safety of you and your baby, it is worth repeating. Note that not all potentially danger-ous foods carry the same degree of risk, so I have categorized the foods here as either "Don't eat" or "Be careful" based on their risk.

Don't Eat

The following foods should *not* be eaten while pregnant as they may pose high risks to you and your baby.

Unpasteurized Milk and Cheeses
You may have heard that all soft cheeses are off-limits during pregnancy. How-ever, it's the pasteurization that really matters. You can indulge in any soft cheese, as long as it's made from pasteurized milk (be sure to check the label; if it doesn't say *pasteurized,* do not eat it). All unpasteurized milk and milk products such as cheese, fresh or frozen yogurt, pudding, and ice cream should be avoided during these nine months. Fortunately, most milk products in the grocery store are pasteurized.

Why the big fuss about pasteurization? Because of a nasty little bug called *Listeria*. While it may only give you a bad case of diarrhea if you're not pregnant and in good health (although it can be lethal, especially in those with weakened immune systems such as newborns and the elderly, and cases of death have been recorded), getting listeriosis during pregnancy can have detrimental effects on your baby. Listeriosis is pretty rare in the general population, but it is ten times more common in women who are pregnant, and 16 to 27 percent of all infections with *Listeria* occur in pregnant women. Although the symptoms of listeriosis may be mild for the mother (flulike symptoms, including fever, backache, headache, vomiting and diarrhea, muscle pains, and sore throat, or even no symptoms at all), it can potentially be lethal to the baby, with 29 percent of all *Listeria* infections during pregnancy ending in miscarriage, stillbirth, or neonatal deaths. In addition to *Listeria*, unpasteurized milk can contain other dangerous bacteria such as *E. coli, Campylobacter,* and *Salmonella*. Listeria infections are the third most deadly foodborne illness (salmonellosis and toxoplasmosis are first and second, respectively).

Due to these health concerns, you should steer clear of raw milk, unpasteurized feta, unpasteurized blue cheeses, unpasteurized Brie, unpasteurized Camembert, unpasteurized queso blanco, unpasteurized queso fresco, unpasteurized panela, other unpasteurized soft cheeses, and any other unpasteurized milk products. If you're unsure whether or not it's pasteurized because nothing is stated on the package or you never saw the package because the cheese was part of a dish served at a restaurant or a party, avoid it and go for something else instead.

NEW PASTEURIZATION LEGISLATION

Over the years, legislation has been passed to ban the sale of unpasteurized milk and milk products, decreasing the chances that this will be much of a problem. However, you can never be too cautious; be sure to check on food labels and ask at restaurants or farmers' markets to ensure that a product is made using pasteurized milk. Similarly, you cannot purchase unpasteurized soft cheeses in major food stores. However, even though you may be less likely to come by unpasteurized soft cheese, it's still available to some extent, so risk of consuming it remains. Unpasteurized *hard* cheeses are a different story, though, and most are freely available in stores and restaurants. However, the FDA requires that they be aged for at least 60 days, which virtually eliminates the risk of listeriosis.

Raw or Undercooked Fish and Seafood

Listeria can also contaminate sushi and other raw fish or seafood. Thus the Centers for Disease Control recommends that all pregnant women avoid consuming sushi and cook all fish to at least 145°F. Because cooking fish or other animal products to optimal temperatures can decrease your risk, it may be helpful to invest in a food thermometer to use during cooking, if you don't have one yet. Similarly, avoid eating raw shellfish, as it can contain *Vibrio* bacteria.

Raw Eggs

Cookie dough ice cream may be on your list of pregnancy food cravings, but watch out. Due to the salmonella that can be present in uncooked eggs, batter, or raw cookie dough, make sure not to lick your fingers or the spoon before baking these, no matter how tempting. Be sure the yolks in cooked eggs are firm (never runny!) and that any foods containing eggs (such as casseroles) are cooked to at least 160°F. And that tempting cookie dough ice cream? Good news! Most store-bought brands don't use raw eggs.

Fish High in Mercury

While the recommendation throughout pregnancy is to consume 12 ounces of fish per week (approximately two meals), you should avoid certain fish because they are high in mercury and may be high in other contaminants as well. Examples of fish with high methylmercury levels are swordfish, tilefish (golden or white snapper), shark, marlin, king mackerel, largemouth bass, larger species of tuna, northern pike, and orange roughy. Additionally, limit your consumption of albacore tuna to 6 ounces per week (a typical can is 5 ounces).

The U.S. Environmental Protection Agency (EPA) periodically releases guidelines about fish that may contain various environmental contaminants, and you can check www.epa.gov/mercury/advisories.htm for the latest updates. In addition, the Natural Resources Defense Council provides reports and lists of fish to avoid and those you can safely consume, based on research regarding the amount of contaminants found. You can access the most recently updated information at www.nrdc.org/health/effects/mercury/guide.asp. It may also be a good idea to have a snapshot of this list on your smartphone so you can access it while in a restaurant to make sure that you order the types of fish that are healthy for you and your baby. Five of the most commonly eaten fish that are low in mercury (and therefore good choices) are salmon, shrimp, canned light tuna, catfish, and pollock.

Raw or Undercooked Sprouts

Sprouts—including alfalfa, radish, mung bean, and clover sprouts—may contain *E. coli* or salmonella, so be sure to cook them to at least 145°F instead of eating them raw.

Liver Products and Supplements Containing Vitamin A

While vitamin A is beneficial and essential throughout pregnancy, too much of it can do more harm than good. Animal liver products can contain very high vitamin A levels, so it is best to avoid them. In addition, you should not take any vitamin A supplements, as this vitamin is naturally contained in a variety of foods, and deficiencies in the developed world are very rare.

Be Careful

Your intake of the following foods should be limited while you're pregnant to avoid risks to you and your baby.

Some Types of Meat, Fish, and Poultry

Similar to unpasteurized milk and milk products, certain types of meat (deli meats, luncheon meats, cold cuts, fermented or dry sausages, and hot dogs) can harbor *Listeria*. Unless they are heated to 165°F or served steaming hot, it is best to avoid them. Also try to avoid getting the fluid from inside hot dog and lunch meat packages onto other foods and surfaces, so that if *Listeria* are present they don't contaminate your other food or kitchen. *Listeria* can also contaminate other processed meats and seafood, like pâtés or meat spreads and refrigerated smoked seafood. Therefore, try to avoid refrigerated pâté or meat spreads from a meat counter or deli, as well as from the refrigerated section of a store. Canned or shelf-stable pâtés and meat spreads that do not require refrigeration are safe to eat—just remember to refrigerate them after opening. Refrigerated smoked seafood, such as cod, mackerel, salmon, trout, tuna, or whitefish, are also potential *Listeria* reservoirs that you might encounter at your local deli or bagel shop. Watch out for labels such as "jerky," "kippered," "lox," "nova-style," or "smoked." Not all processed seafood products are off-limits, however; canned and shelf-stable fish (such as salmon, tuna, and others) and fish products, as well as cooked, smoked fish dishes such as casseroles, are all safe and perfectly fine to eat.

The meat, poultry, or seafood in ready-to-eat salads can also harbor *Listeria*. We like to have faith in eating establishments, but you really don't know whether meats have been properly cooked, and even if they have, they may have come into contact with parts and pieces of food that haven't been adequately cooked, thus getting contaminated upon contact. And while you can heat up deli meats and cold cuts to eliminate any potential *Listeria* (that's why they're in the "Be careful" section instead of the "Don't eat" section), you can't do that with a salad.

Your best bet is to make your own chicken or tuna salad at home, following safe food handling and preparation instructions. And when you are out at a restaurant, it can't hurt to ask the server for your chicken or other meat to be cooked "very well done." Finally, while meat, fish, and poultry all provide vitamins and nutrients that you and your baby need, it's important to make sure they don't pose any health risks. Undercooked fish may contain bacteria or parasites, undercooked meat may contain *E. coli,* and undercooked poultry can carry *Campylobacter* or *Salmonella.* Because of these concerns, be sure to cook all fish and meat to 145°F and all ground meat, pork, and poultry to 165°F to kill any potential bacteria.

General Recommendations to Prevent an Infection with Listeria

Rinse	Raw produce, such as fruits and veggies, thoroughly under running tap water before eating, cutting, or cooking. Even if the produce will be peeled, you should still wash it first.
Scrub	Firm produce, such as melons and cucumbers, with a clean produce brush
Dry	The produce with either a clean cloth or paper towel
Separate	Uncooked meats and poultry from veggies, cooked foods, and ready-to-eat foods
Wash	Hands, knives, countertops, and cutting boards after handling and preparing uncooked foods with hot water and soap
Clean up	All spills in your fridge right away—especially juices from lunch/hot dog meat packages, raw meats, and poultry
Cool	Listeria can grow even in foods that are in the fridge. Make sure that your refrigerator is at 40°F or lower at all times, and the freezer is at 0°F or lower
Store	Unused food as soon as you're done eating. Choose shallow containers to promote rapid, even cooling. Cover with airtight lids or enclose in plastic wrap or aluminum foil. Use all leftovers within 3 or 4 days, and never store or use precooked or ready-to-eat foods beyond the use-by date.

Source: Centers for Disease Control (CDC), Listeria (Listeriosis) Prevention *(2013). Available at www.cdc.gov/listeria/prevention.html. Accessed July 10, 2014.*

Cantaloupe

Cantaloupe is a recent addition to the list, due to the biggest outbreak of *Listeria*, in September 2011, when *Listeria* contamination of cantaloupes (from a single farm) affected 147 people in 28 states, leading to 33 deaths and 1 miscarriage. Should you now avoid eating melons while pregnant? No. But you should wash your hands with warm water and soap for at least 20 seconds before and after handling any melons, including watermelon, cantaloupe, or honeydew. Before cutting, you should also scrub the rind of the melon with a clean produce brush under running water and dry it with a clean paper towel. Last, you should consume the melon promptly after cutting (discard the melon if it's been out at room temperature for more than 4 hours) and refrigerate leftovers at 40°F or lower (32° to 34°F is best) for no more than 7 days. If you purchase cut and wrapped melon halves or wedges, be sure to thoroughly wash them.

A QUICK WORD ABOUT FRESH PRODUCE

You do not need to avoid fresh produce during pregnancy by any means; on the contrary, try to consume lots of it. However, make sure you wash and scrub your fruits and veggies thoroughly with a brush under running water (don't use soap) before cutting and eating them. This will help reduce the potential risk of toxoplasmosis. The *Toxoplasma* parasite can live on unwashed fruits and veggies, and if consumed, can pose serious risks to your baby.

Controversial Foods and Beverages: What Recent Research Shows

You may have doubts about some of the foods and drinks you are advised not to consume during pregnancy. You may be thinking, *Can it really cause that much harm?* or *What if I have just a little bit?* Let's look at what the research suggests regarding alcohol, coffee, herbal teas, and peanut consumption during pregnancy.

Alcohol

Alcohol is a well-known teratogen, meaning that it can cause malformations and abnormalities in a developing baby. Numerous studies have reported hundreds of negative health outcomes due to maternal drinking, ranging from fetal alcohol syndrome spectrum abnormalities to increased risk of ADHD, heart defects, poor memory, and many others. But is it true that you can't have *any* alcohol during pregnancy? What about all the French and Italian women who enjoy a glass of red wine regardless of their growing baby? The truth is, alcohol consumption can be highly detrimental to your baby, but it depends on how much, how often, and when in the pregnancy alcohol is consumed.

The embryonic stage, or the first 8 weeks of pregnancy, is the most sensitive period, and you should be particularly careful during this time. However, the first 2 weeks following fertilization is when implantation occurs, and while alcohol probably does not help the process, research shows that it does not have a particularly harmful effect on the zygote. Still, alcohol consumed during this time may lead to miscarriage—possibly before you even know that you are pregnant. If you did consume alcohol at the time of conception and for up to 2 weeks afterward and did not miscarry, however, it is likely that your baby was not harmed by it. It is in the third week post-fertilization that drinking alcohol really starts to matter. This is when the three embryonic germ layers are set and your baby's nervous system starts to develop. In weeks 4, 5, 6, 7, and 8, your baby's organs and organ systems are forming at a fast pace, and drinking alcohol at this time is very risky, as it can lead to organ-specific abnormalities, fetal alcohol syndrome (FAS), and even miscarriage if alcohol damage is too severe. And although FAS is the most severe form of alcohol-related birth defects, drinking in the first 8 weeks of pregnancy can lead to many other consequences that may not be as severe as FAS but still impact your child's health. A recent study looking at alcohol consumption prior to and during pregnancy found that the first trimester was the most sensitive in terms of detrimental effects of alcohol, leading to increased risk of low birth weight and preterm birth. Researchers concluded that all women should abstain from drinking throughout pregnancy.

After the eighth week, because most of the organ systems have been established by this time, the effects of alcohol may not be as severe, even though it still has the potential to negatively impact normal development. An important thing to keep in mind, however, is that your baby's brain continues to develop until birth, so alcohol consumption at any point in the pregnancy may have an impact on neural development and mental health. In general, even though drinking in the first 8 weeks is known to have more serious consequences than drinking later in pregnancy, there is no point in pregnancy when alcohol exposure is entirely without potential harm to your baby.

Does the research say anything in alcohol's defense? A study looking at intelligence, attention, and executive function of 5-year-old children whose mothers consumed alcohol in low (1 to 4 drinks per week) or moderate (5 to

8 drinks per week) amounts early on and up to mid-pregnancy found no difference between these children and those whose mothers abstained from any alcohol use, suggesting that alcohol consumed occasionally may not confer serious risk with respect to these variables. Additionally, a recent review of studies looking at the effects of low to moderate drinking during pregnancy on children's speech and language abilities could neither confirm nor deny that alcohol had any effect.

My recommendation falls into the conservative category of abstaining from alcohol throughout pregnancy, although I do believe that a sip of wine in the second or third trimester is unlikely to have a significant impact on your baby's health. I err on the side of caution for two main reasons. First, even though some studies show no association between mild or moderate alcohol consumption at some points during the pregnancy and any ill effects on the baby, no study has looked at every possible health outcome in relation to drinking alcohol, leaving some questions unanswered. Furthermore, although there are no visible differences in, for example, attention span or intelligence at age 5 does not mean there won't be differences at age 15, 30, or 70.

Coffee and Tea

Whether or not women should give up or restrict coffee consumption during pregnancy has been up for debate for a while now, and the research is still inconsistent regarding its safety for your baby. A study conducted with Danish women found no difference in terms of birth weight, preterm birth, or growth restriction between women who were randomly assigned to either drink up to 3 cups of caffeinated or up to 3 cups of decaffeinated coffee per day. Similarly, analyses of studies on caffeine intake during pregnancy found no detrimental effects on the risk of preterm birth, congenital malformations, miscarriage, or growth retardation. There is, however, some evidence that high consumption of coffee can be detrimental, and research-based evidence suggests that women limit caffeine consumption from all foods and beverages to 200 to 300 mg or less per day. This translates to 1 to 3 cups of coffee per day, depending on how strong it's brewed. It is important to remember that caffeine is not found only in tea and coffee; it is also present in sodas, chocolate, and other sources, such as certain kinds of chewing gum. Therefore, if you are a coffee drinker, try to moderate your coffee consumption to 3 cups or less per day, and 0 to 2 cups if you also consume chocolate, soda, or other caffeine products on any particular day.

Raw Juice

Unfortunately, unless you make it yourself, you never know how thoroughly someone else cleaned (or didn't clean) fruits and veggies before juicing them, thus putting you and your baby at risk for contracting a foodborne illness due to the *Toxoplasma* and other bacteria that can be present on unwashed or improperly cleaned produce. Some delis and restaurants offer freshly juiced raw juices, but I would advise against drinking them, because in addition to not knowing how carefully they were prepared, you don't know how long they've been sitting there. Even if it has been only a few hours, that's sufficient time for bacteria to grow and multiply and increase your risk for food poisoning. Fortunately, you can juice all you want if you're doing it yourself. There is currently no research indicating that drinking juice you make yourself when pregnant is harmful if you follow safe food handling guidelines and drink it promptly. So juice as much (or as little) as you want, but make sure to properly wash and scrub your produce under running water with a brush to get rid of any possible bugs that can cause harm. You may also want to use soap on certain fruits, such as oranges or grapefruit, to remove any germs or pesticides that may be on their surface, as those can get into the fruit (and fruit juice) once you cut them. In addition to juicing, you can make smoothies; this can add some fiber to your diet, which becomes increasingly important with every week of pregnancy due to constipation.

Herbal Teas

Some herbal teas may be beneficial during pregnancy, as they contain valuable vitamins and minerals. Others are considered less safe because they may not actually contain everything the label says and they are still poorly regulated. It is best to consult your health care provider about drinking any herbal teas during pregnancy, especially if you plan to drink them regularly. He or she may be able to recommend a particular brand or variety known to be safe and use clinical judgment and expertise in advising you, based on experience with prenatal use of herbs.

Because there are hundreds of herbal teas and covering all of them is beyond the scope of this book, I encourage anyone who is interested in learning more about the safety and potential benefits of herbal teas to look at the American Pregnancy Association ratings (from the Natural Medicines Database) at Americanpregnancy.org.

Peanuts and Tree Nuts

Peanut and tree nut consumption in pregnancy has been controversial for years, as some people think it may increase the risk of peanut and tree nut allergies in children. However, recent research doesn't support this claim. A large-scale study involving nearly sixty-two thousand pregnant women showed no adverse outcomes (including no increase in nut allergies) and found a decreased risk of asthma in children of mothers who reported eating peanuts one or more times per week. Another large study that recorded pregnant women's diets and followed both them and their children for 10 to 15 years afterward found that higher consumption of peanuts and tree nuts by mothers before, during, and after pregnancy (five or more times per month) actually decreased the risk of peanut and tree nut allergies in their children. The current guideline is that pregnant women *do not* have to avoid peanuts, tree nuts, or any other potential allergens (such as fish, eggs, milk, and others) unless they themselves are allergic to these foods. So feel free to go nuts! Just remember that like all nuts, peanuts and tree nuts are high in calories, so you might want to limit your intake to a few servings per week. However, if you know that you are allergic or suspect that you might be allergic, avoid peanuts and tree nuts by all means, or talk to your health care provider.

* * *

Yikes! That's quite a few foods to avoid or be cautious about, right? Is all this really necessary? The bottom line is that during pregnancy your immune system is weakened, making you more susceptible to almost everything, from the common cold to foodborne illnesses and beyond. The CDC reports that each year one in six Americans get a foodborne illness (that's about 48 million people!), of which 128,000 are hospitalized and 3,000 die. Furthermore, as mentioned earlier, the CDC reports that foodborne infections such as listeriosis disproportionately affect pregnant women. In fact, 90 percent of all people who get listeriosis are pregnant women and their newborns, the elderly, and other people with weakened immune systems. Thus pregnancy is a time of heightened vulnerability, and any efforts you can make to help prevent health problems for yourself or your baby by avoiding certain foods and beverages are always encouraged.

Appendix B: Eating Well While Nursing

Eating a balanced diet and maintaining adequate calorie intake while nursing are essential for both your and your baby's health, as well as for optimal milk supply. What you eat while breastfeeding will affect the amount of some (but not all) of the nutrients in your milk, and therefore the amount of nutrients your baby gets, as breast milk may be the sole source of nourishment for your little one. In addition, your diet and how long you breastfeed (6 months, 1 year, and so on) can impact your own health as well as your post-pregnancy weight loss. This appendix will provide you with information about some of the benefits of breastfeeding, an overview of the nutrients contained in breast milk, and what to eat to ensure optimal breast milk composition.

The Benefits of Breastfeeding for You and Your Baby

The benefits of breastfeeding are vast, leading many health care providers to argue that it is the best thing you can do for your baby's—and your own—health. Nicknamed "liquid gold," human milk is an amazing and all-natural nutritional substance. If you are on the fence about it, here are a few points that may provide you with some encouragement:

- Breastfeeding has been associated with lower infant morbidity (disease or illness) and mortality (death) as well as better long-term health.

- Breastfeeding has been shown to lead to a higher intelligence quotient (IQ) in many studies, with an association between the duration of breastfeeding and increase in IQ points at ages 7 to 8. Breastfeeding has also been shown to have long-term effects on cognitive development, with higher IQs in adults who were breastfed compared to those who were not, and higher IQs with greater duration of breastfeeding.

- Risk of sudden infant death syndrome (SIDS) is lower in breastfed infants.

- Breastfed infants have lower rates of the following chronic diseases in later life compared to those who were not breastfed: juvenile diabetes, obesity, food allergies, atopic dermatitis, celiac disease, Crohn's disease, ulcerative colitis, lymphoma, and malocclusion.

- Breastfed infants are less likely to develop childhood diseases such as asthma, childhood obesity, and otitis media (ear infection), or get rotavirus and respiratory infections such as bronchopneumonia and bronchiolitis.

- Breastfed infants are less likely to be hospitalized for lower respiratory tract disease in the first year of life.

- Breastfeeding protects the baby from an excess of protein and may reduce the overall risk of obesity much later in life. Formula-fed infants get 70 percent more protein than breastfed infants; the excess protein causes increased production of insulin and insulin growth factor-1, which can result in increased weight gain by 2 years of age and increased fat tissue production, and may send them down a course for greater weight in later life.

- Breastfeeding can reduce a mother's risk of ovarian and breast cancer and possibly the risk of hip fractures and osteoporosis after menopause.

- Breastfeeding may help lower the risk of postpartum depression.

HIGHLY RECOMMENDED

Because breastfeeding has many health and psychosocial benefits, it is widely recommended by numerous prominent organizations of health professionals, such as the following:

The World Health Organization

American Academy of Pediatrics

American Academy of Family Physicians

American Congress of Obstetricians and Gynecologists

American College of Nurse-Midwives

American Dietetic Association

American Public Health Association

All of these organizations recommend exclusive breastfeeding for the first 6 months (meaning that infants should not be given any foods or liquids other than breast milk, not even water), and breast-feeding for at least 12 months, with supplementary foods introduced at 6 months of age. Again, these are just guidelines, and your pediatrician may have other advice based on your baby's specific needs.

All of that said, remember that breastfeeding isn't for everyone. For some women (like me), medical complications after delivery can prohibit breastfeeding. Others may try it and, rather than the blissful picture that most of us envision, find that it ends up being stressful and causes tears (from both you and the baby!). Others may just not want to do it, just because they don't want to. That's fine! If you don't breastfeed your baby, for whatever reason, don't waste time feeling guilty or rethinking your choice. Having a happy mommy is more important to your baby, and your baby will be just fine.

How Many Calories Do You Need While Breastfeeding?

Just as you did during the second and third trimesters, you also need some extra calories during the lactation period. In fact, you need even more than during pregnancy: about 500 extra calories daily. That's roughly how many calories your body has to expend daily to make enough milk for your baby.

Five hundred extra calories may sound like a feast, but just as you did with the extra calories during pregnancy, aim to "spend" them on wholesome, nutrient-dense foods. Fruits, vegetables, whole grains, lean proteins, and low-fat dairy products are all excellent sources to obtain the extra energy you need.

500 CALORIES

What does 500 calories look like? The extra calories you need during nursing are roughly equal to one extra meal or several snacks consumed throughout the day. The following are some examples of foods that are about equal to 500 calories.

1 cup of plain low-fat yogurt (143 calories), 1 medium-size banana (105 calories), 1 tablespoon of peanut butter (95 calories), 1 glass of orange juice (117 calories), and 4 ounces of raw baby carrots (40 calories)

3 ounces of grilled salmon (118 calories), 1 cup of cooked lentils (226 calories), 1 cup of roasted brussels sprouts (56 calories), 2 ounces of raw baby kale (28 calories), and ⅓ ounce of raw walnuts (62 calories)

What Is in My Breast Milk and How Does My Diet Affect It?

Breast milk contains all the vitamins, minerals, macronutrients, and calories that your baby needs for the first 6 months of life in the correct proportions (with the exception of vitamins D and K). The composition of breast milk varies from feed to feed, between mothers, by gestational age, and throughout the duration of lactation (at 1 month, 6 months, and so on); it even differs based on time of the day as well as the length of the feed (the composition of *foremilk*, which is the milk you produce at the beginning of a feeding, is higher in fat than that of *hindmilk*, the milk you produce at the end of a feeding).

Your own diet also has an impact on the contents of your milk and can particularly affect its taste and smell. For example, your baby will know if you had spicy curry for dinner, as your breast milk will contain some of the flavors of the spices that you had in your meal. Similarly, some of the flavors from the fruits and vegetables that you eat will seep into your milk, and your baby will experience them. By being exposed to a variety of flavors early on, your baby is learning about these different tastes and smells and later on may be more likely to choose to eat those foods. In fact, studies show that breastfed infants are less picky, more willing to try new foods, and consume more fruits and vegetables in childhood compared to formula-fed babies. Therefore, it is very important to consume a wholesome and varied diet while breastfeeding, because not only will your baby be consuming what you eat, by extension, but also it may influence your child's food choices and, in turn, health later in life.

YOUR NUTRITIONAL STATE DURING PREGNANCY CAN AFFECT YOUR NUTRITIONAL STATUS DURING LACTATION

While you can make up for any nutrient insufficiencies or deficiencies after your baby is born, it is best to avoid them and ensure optimal intake of all nutrients during the nine months before lactation. If your body stores are lacking one nutrient or another while you're pregnant, at least at the very beginning of lactation your baby will be getting less of that nutrient in the breast milk. For example, a study that compared the breast milk of women who received an EPA and DHA supplements during pregnancy with those who did not found that the levels of EPA and DHA at day 3 and week 6 after delivery were higher in the women who supplemented. In addition, the levels of DHA in the baby at 1 year of age were directly related to the DHA levels in the mother's milk at day 3 and week 6, and the babies of mothers who were supplemented (and thus had higher milk levels of EPA and DHA) had better developmental scores at 2.5 years of age, including better eye and hand coordination.

The content of some nutrients in your milk is sensitive to your diet and may be less than optimal if your diet is lacking them. The concentrations of vitamins A, C, D, B1, B2, B3, B6, and B12, fatty acids, and iodine in your milk are influenced by your diet, whereas calories, folate, minerals, and trace elements are not. However, your intake of the latter nutrients still needs to be higher compared to nonbreastfeeding women so that your own body stores do not get depleted in the process. Note that, similar to your caloric needs, your needs for some vitamins, minerals, and macronutrients are even higher during lactation than they were during pregnancy. See the table on pages 186–187 for the nutrients you'll need in greater amounts during lactation.

Just as when you were pregnant, you don't need to stress about getting the exact amount of each nutrient every day; as long as your *average* intake over the course of several days is adequate, your nutritional status and the nutrient content of your breast milk will be okay. In addition, despite all the numbers for each nutrient that are given in the table, do not worry too much about your intake of any one food or nutrient; instead, focus on getting a regular, balanced diet. As I briefly mentioned before, some of the nutrients in your milk are not even affected by your diet, and the ones that are influenced by what you eat can be easily obtained (from foods that you may already be eating regularly). Furthermore, some of the factors that do have an effect on your milk composition are somewhat beyond your control. A study in California, for example, found that in addition to protein intake, factors such as maternal BMI, number of children, return of menstruation, and nursing frequency were all associated with macronutrient concentrations of breast milk.

Breastfeeding Superfoods

While a wholesome, balanced, and varied diet is always the main goal, some foods are particularly beneficial during breastfeeding, as they are densely packed with the nutrients that are important at this time and that have an impact on your milk composition (vitamins A, B1, B2, B3, B6, B12, C, D, iodine, and fatty acids). It is a good idea to incorporate them into your diet if you are not doing so already.

continued on page 188

Nutritional Needs during Lactation

Nutrient	Amount Needed Daily during Lactation	Amount Needed during Pregnancy	Food Sources
Calcium	1,000 mg	1,000 mg	Milk, yogurt, turnip greens, kale, fortified orange juice and fortified breakfast cereals, calcium-set tofu, collard greens
Carbohydrate	210 g	175 g	Fruits and vegetables, whole wheat cereals, pasta, bread
Choline	450 mg	450 mg	Wheat germ, broccoli, tofu, quinoa, milk, spinach, eggs, potatoes, chicken, navy and soybeans, fish, nuts
EPA and DHA	350 mg EPA, 300 mg DHA	350 mg EPA; 300 mg DHA	Salmon, catfish, canned light tuna, anchovies, herring, halibut, fish oil, fortified eggs
Fiber	29 g	28 g	Whole grains, lentils, beans, vegetables, fruit
Folate	500 DFE	600 DFE	Spinach, kale, boiled kidney beans, lentils
Iodine	290 mcg	220 mcg	Iodized salt, iodized milk and bread (in the U.S.)
Iron	9 mg	27 mg	Meats, fish, seafood, poultry, fortified cereals, eggs, milk, pumpkin seeds, lentils and other legumes, spinach, prune juice
Magnesium	310 mg (19–30 yrs old) 320 mg (31–50 yrs old)	350 mg (19–30 yrs old) 360 mg (31–50 yrs old)	Pumpkin and sunflower seeds, salmon, halibut, wheat germ, bran cereal, quinoa, brown rice, almonds, cashews, soybeans, spinach, tofu, baked potato (with skin)
Phosphorus	700 mg	700 mg	Yogurt, milk, cheese, fish, poultry, nuts, eggs, cereals
Potassium	5.1 g	4.7 g	Baked sweet potato, plain yogurt, milk, nuts and seeds, kale, lentils, banana, orange juice, winter squash
Protein	1.1 g per kg of body weight	1.1 g per kg of body weight	Milk, cheese, egg whites, soybeans, rice, quinoa, beef, chickpeas, black beans, fruits, vegetables, legumes

Nutrient	Amount Needed Daily during Lactation	Amount Needed during Pregnancy	Food Sources
Vitamin A	1,300 mcg	770 mcg	Carrots, eggs, kale, oatmeal, cantaloupe, spinach, sweet potato, cheese
Vitamin B1	1.4 mg	1.4 mg	Meats (pork, poultry), fish, fortified breads and cereals, nuts and seeds, beans
Vitamin B2	1.6 mg	1.4 mg	Milk, cheese, yogurt, ice cream, almonds, meats, fish, eggs, mushrooms, spinach
Vitamin B3	17 mg	18 mg	Eggs, fish, meat, poultry, peanuts, milk, mushrooms, avocado, green peas, sun-flower seeds
Vitamin B6	2 mg	1.9 mg	Baked potato, salmon, chicken, cooked spinach, prune juice, chickpeas, brown rice, banana, avocado, pork loin
Vitamin B12	2.8 mcg	2.6 mcg	Beef, cod, salmon, milk, cheese, eggs
Vitamin C	120 mg	85 mg	Oranges, broccoli, guava, papaya, bell peppers (yellow, green, red), sweet potato, mango, brussels sprouts, kiwifruit
Vitamin D	600 IU (15 mcg)	600 IU (15 mcg)	Fatty fish (salmon, trout), fortified milk and orange juice, egg yolks
Vitamin K	90 mcg	90 mcg	Leafy greens: kale, collards, spinach, cabbage, mustard greens, Swiss chard, brussels sprouts
Zinc	12 mg	11 mg	Ground beef, turkey, Alaskan king crab, tofu, pumpkin seeds, garbanzo and kidney beans, whole grains, milk, collard greens

- **Lentils.** A "food of the week" during the first trimester of pregnancy, lentils are also an excellent source of nutrients during lactation. They are loaded with lean protein, complex carbohydrates, potassium, folate, and fiber and contain moderate amounts of vitamins B1, B2, B3, and B6.

- **Kale.** This leafy green is invaluable during lactation, especially because of its high vitamin A, C, and K content, and moderate amounts of the B vitamins.

- **Pineapple.** High in vitamin C, pineapple can be a great milk "sweetener" and give your baby early exposure to a delicious and healthy fruit.

- **Wild salmon.** The goldmine of omega-3s, salmon should be eaten on a regular basis to get some EPA and DHA into your milk. As I mentioned before, EPA and DHA levels in breast milk (especially early on) will be affected by your diet while pregnant, but your dietary intake of these and other omega-3s during lactation will continue to affect the levels in your milk. Your baby's brain will continue developing rapidly from birth until 2 years of age (and later as well, but the most rapid growth will occur by age 2), and omega-3s are essential to support healthy brain development. Studies show that babies of women who consume 8 to 12 ounces of low-mercury fish per week have better visual and cognitive development than those who don't. In case that's not enough to sway you toward the seafood section of the supermarket, wild salmon also contains plenty of vitamins D and B12 (one serving has nearly twice the recommended daily amount of vitamin B12 and more than half of the daily recommendation for vitamin D), B3, and moderate amounts of other B vitamins. Finally, your milk is sensitive to salmon's mono- and polyunsaturated fatty acids, which are also crucial for your baby's developing brain.

- **Sweet pepper (yellow, red, orange).** Packed with vitamins A and C, sweet peppers will not only enrich your milk with these crucial nutrients but also expose your baby to this veggie early on, potentially increasing the odds that baby will reach for these veggies later on in childhood— and adulthood.

- **Water.** While water is undoubtedly a part of your diet already, make sure you are getting plenty of it during the breastfeeding period. Ninety percent of your breast milk is water, so keep yourself well hydrated at all times. The recommended amount for women who are breastfeeding is 3.8 liters (roughly 16 cups) of water per day, which is a *lot*. Focus on listening to your body, and keep a glass or bottle of water handy at all times (you can also drink water while breastfeeding). Try not to wait until you feel thirsty; keep sipping water throughout the day. However, don't overdo it either, as that may cause discomfort.

Now That I'm No Longer Pregnant (But Nursing), Can I . . .

There were several activities that you had to graciously bow out of while pregnant. And now that you are no longer carrying a baby in your belly, you are probably wondering whether you can resume your usual activities. Read on.

Drink Alcohol?

Good news, mama: you can now enjoy a glass of wine here and there without the added stress of how it may affect your baby as it develops in the womb! However, you cannot drink to the same extent as a woman who is not breastfeeding. In fact, the conservative recommendation is to completely abstain from alcohol until you are no longer breastfeeding. That said, a couple of glasses of wine per week are A-okay—just be sure to exercise caution. If you choose to have a drink, do so right after a feed, so that about 4 hours pass before the next feeding and your body metabolizes the alcohol (the alcohol content of your breast milk is similar to that of your blood). More hours are needed if you have more than one drink, so it may be a good idea to limit yourself to just one, or alternatively, plan ahead—pump before drinking and store the milk in advance so that you're not faced with the dilemma of a hungry, crying baby and only alcoholic milk to feed it. Additionally, you can screen your milk for alcohol before breastfeeding with a simple test (such as Milkscreen, a home test for the presence of alcohol in breast milk) that will tell you whether there's any residual alcohol left in your milk, because to date no level of alcohol in breast milk has been determined safe for a baby.

BABY COMES FIRST ────────────────────────────

You should not consume *any* amount of alcohol before your baby develops consistent latch on and breastfeeding patterns.

Research on the long-term effects of alcohol consumption during the breastfeeding period is still limited, but the current data show that in the short term, alcohol inhibits lactation and the milk ejection reflex, which may some-what reduce your milk supply—something to keep in mind, especially if your milk supply is already on the low side. While long-term consequences are unknown, so far occasional drinking while breastfeeding has not been con-vincingly shown to adversely affect nursing infants. The bottom line: remem-ber that moderation is key, and check your milk for alcohol before a feeding. It's always better to be safe than sorry—and keep some pumped breast milk stored, in case you test positive and baby is hungry.

HOW MUCH IS ONE DRINK?

"One drink" is not necessarily the amount you pour into your glass. It is defined as:

- 340 g (12 ounces) of 5% beer, or

- 141.75 g (5 ounces) of 11% wine, or

- 42.53 g (1.5 ounces) of 40% liquor

Use a measuring cup because eyeballing it isn't very accurate.

Drink Coffee?

Just like during pregnancy, moderation is key; drinking up to 2 or 3 cups a day is fine for your baby. Also, keep in mind that foods other than coffee can contain caffeine (soda, tea, chocolate, chewing gum, and others), so be sure to read food labels to avoid excessive intake.

Eat High-Mercury Fish?

Similar to when you were pregnant, try your best to steer clear of all high-mercury fish. If you eat these, the methylmercury and other pollutants and heavy metals present in these fish will get into your milk and will thus be passed on to your baby, increasing the risk of neurodevelopmental issues. Studies have shown delays in the age of walking and talking, as well as lower mental and psychomotor development index scores, in infants exposed to mercury, lead, and methylmercury in breast milk.

Raw Fish and Shellfish, Sprouts, Juice, and Everything Else?

Unlike during pregnancy, your immune system is no longer suppressed, so you can return to many of the food habits you've been avoiding. Sushi is now fine to consume, as long as it doesn't contain any high-mercury fish. In addition, everything else that you may have been consuming before getting pregnant—such as raw juice, raw shellfish, deli meats, raw sprouts, and other raw or unpasteurized foods—are now fine to eat. That said, you should continue to exercise regular safe food handling techniques to lower any risk of food poisoning.

Appendix C: Special Medical Considerations

There are certain conditions that women may have when entering pregnancy or that can develop during a pregnancy that may require special medical and dietary attention. When expecting, women may experience high blood pressure, preeclampsia, and gestational diabetes, all of which may require special nutritional interventions to help decrease the risks associated with these conditions. Additionally, increased nutritional requirements are suggested for women expecting twins. In this appendix, I give an overview of the most common conditions that can occur during pregnancy and provide nutritional advice that can help reduce your risk of complications or support your pregnancy with multiples.

HIGH BLOOD PRESSURE DEFINED ————————————

High blood pressure is defined as a systolic blood pressure of at least 140 mm Hg and a diastolic blood pressure of at least 90 mm Hg. Blood pressure figures are usually stated as systolic/diastolic, such as 140/90.

Gestational High Blood Pressure and Preeclampsia

More common in overweight and obese mothers, gestational hypertension (high blood pressure during pregnancy) affects about 6 to 17 percent of first-time mothers and 2 to 5 percent of non-first-time mothers. About half of all women with gestational hypertension diagnosed before 30 weeks of gestation go on to develop preeclampsia, a more severe form of hypertension that is associated with increased risk of preterm delivery, low birth weight, and neonatal and maternal death, and a greater risk that the mother will develop cardiovascular disease later in life. When you have preeclampsia, your placenta is not working as well as it should, so it is delivering less oxygen and nutrients to your baby, meaning that baby may have less-than-optimal growth while in your belly and may not reach its full developmental potential. Risk factors for preeclampsia include having had preeclampsia in a previous pregnancy, being younger than 20 or older than 40 at the time of pregnancy, having a BMI in the obese range (30 and above), having insulin resistance or diabetes, carrying twins, and having certain genetic factors.

The good news is that there are ways to both reduce your chances of developing preeclampsia and prevent complications in case you have already developed it. First, it is very important not to gain excessive weight during your pregnancy, as obesity and excessive weight gain are some of the biggest risk factors for developing preeclampsia. In the same vein, you should avoid consuming excess calories, calorie-rich foods, and foods high in added sugars. A study examining women's intake of calories, sucrose, and polyunsaturated fatty acids in the second trimester found that those who consumed any of the three in excess had a higher risk of developing preeclampsia compared to those who had moderate intakes. A recent study of first-time mothers in Norway at risk for preeclampsia showed that a high intake of vegetables, plant foods, and vegetable oils decreased the risk, whereas greater consumption of processed meats, sweet drinks, and salty snacks increased the risk. In addition, a review of numerous studies found that calcium supplementation reduced the risk of preeclampsia by approximately half. Further, this reduced the risk of preterm birth and death (especially in high-risk women with previously low calcium intake). Higher vitamin D intake from supplements (but not from diet alone) has also been shown to decrease the risk of preeclampsia by 27 percent in a large cohort of Norwegian women.

Many other vitamins, minerals, nutrients, and foods (including marine-sourced oil, omega-3s, garlic, antioxidants, progesterone, diuretics, nitric oxide, fiber, magnesium, vitamins A, C, and E, folic acid, and other micronutrients) have also been investigated for their effects on preeclampsia, but with conflicting results. Although it is recommended that nonpregnant individuals with high blood pressure limit their sodium intake, along with other dietary modifications, so far this has not been shown to prevent preeclampsia in pregnant women. However, you should still adhere to the 2.3 g per day (or less) recommendation for the general population in order to maintain optimal health. Finally, eating fresh garlic (or taking a garlic supplement) daily has been used in cases of preeclampsia and pregnancy hypertension to lower blood pressure. In one study, taking a 800-mg garlic supplement pill (Garlet) every day during the third trimester of pregnancy reduced the occurrence of hypertension. It did not, however, prevent the development of preeclampsia.

Gestational Diabetes

Gestational diabetes is a type of diabetes that can occur during pregnancy and usually goes away after delivery. Diabetes develops when your body's cells have an abnormal response to insulin (insulin is produced by your pancreas and is the hormone needed for your cells to normally process the glucose that you get from your diet) and fail to convert sugar into energy, resulting in a spike in blood glucose levels. Gestational diabetes affects about 7 percent of all U.S. pregnancies each year and is treated by controlling blood sugar levels, which can be achieved by following a special diet and engaging in regular exercise. Some women, however, need insulin shots or have to take diabetes medication. It is important to treat gestational diabetes, as the condition increases your risk of delivering a macrosomic (9 pounds or heavier) and hypoglycemic (low blood sugar) baby and raises your risk of developing type 2 diabetes later in life.

CAN YOU PREVENT GESTATIONAL DIABETES?

By losing excess weight *before* pregnancy, as well as by following healthy eating guidelines and maintaining a regular physical activity routine both before and during pregnancy, you *can* reduce your risk of developing gestational diabetes. A study looking at the relationship between prepregnancy diet and the risk of gestational diabetes found that a diet with low fiber (low total fiber as well as low fiber from cereals and fruit) and a high glycemic load were associated with an increased risk of developing gestational diabetes. In fact, with each 10 g of total fiber consumed, the risk of developing gestational diabetes decreased by 26 percent, and each 5-g increment in fiber consumption from cereal or fruit was associated with a 23 percent or 26 percent reduction in gestational diabetes risk, respectively.

Even though gestational diabetes is one of the most common pregnancy complications, there remains a lack of consensus regarding the best nutrition management approach. In fact, a recent large-scale Cochrane review of several different diets (low-GI diet, low-moderate GI diet, low-carbohydrate diet, energy-restricted diet, high–monounsaturated fat diet, and high-fiber diet) did not find any particular one to be superior to others in terms of the risk of macrosomia or Cesarean delivery. However, there are certain dietary guidelines for managing gestational diabetes. Keeping your blood glucose levels stable during pregnancy is the main goal, as it has been shown to reduce the risks. If you

what to eat when you're pregnant

develop gestational diabetes during your pregnancy, your doctor will discuss care with you and explain the available medication options as well as the need for regular blood sugar monitoring. In this section, however, I will focus on nutritional therapy for diabetes management and other related approaches that have recently shown promise in treating gestational diabetes; these, combined with regular, moderate physical activity (like walking, swimming, jogging, and weight resistance) will help you achieve and maintain normal blood glucose levels until delivery. To start, here are some dietary adjustments that you can make if you are told you have gestational diabetes.

Manage the Type and Amount of Carbohydrates You Consume Daily

While you need plenty of carbohydrates during pregnancy to supply yourself and your baby with energy, the key now is to ensure that you get your carbohydrates from healthy, nutrient-dense, high-fiber foods, and that you consume them in approximately equal amounts throughout the day. You can get healthy carbohydrates from whole grain, high-fiber, dairy, starchy, and other foods, such as:

- Whole wheat bread, pasta, noodles, whole grain cereals
- Potatoes, legumes
- Quinoa, couscous, buckwheat
- Low-fat milk, yogurt
- Vegetables and fruit

Eat Frequently: You should aim to consume three meals and two to four snacks each day. That means eating every 2.5 to 3 hours. In addition, you should aim to consume about the same amount of carbohydrates with every meal and snack, for a total of about twelve or more servings of carbohydrate per day (one serving equals 15 g of carbohydrate). The total energy that you get from carbs should be less than half of all the calories you consume. (For example, if you consume 2,000 calories per day, less than 1,000 should come from carbohydrates. One gram of carbohydrate equals approximately 4 calories, meaning that your carbohydrate intake should not exceed roughly 250 g per day.) However, do not go on a low-carb diet and limit your carbohydrate intake so that it falls below the 175 g/day recommendation. Remember that carbohydrates are essential for both you and your baby, so make sure you get enough—just aim for the healthy ones and eat them at regular intervals.

Don't Skip Meals: Consuming foods at regular intervals and with similar levels of carbohydrates will help keep your blood glucose levels in a normal range, without sharp drops or spikes, which is the goal of gestational diabetes management.

Choose Healthy Fats: Healthy fats are those from plant and fish foods (avocado, salmon, nuts); try to avoid too much of the "bad" saturated fats that are typically found in butter, cheese, hamburgers, junk food, fried foods, and others. A recent study found that gestational diabetes is associated with high energy (calories) and high saturated fat intakes during pregnancy, regardless of prepregnancy BMI, so try to avoid consuming an excess of the "bad" fats and an excess of total energy (calories).

Know the Glycemic Index (GI) of Different Foods: While research on the effects of low-GI foods in terms of preventing gestational diabetes complications is still mixed, some studies show that for women who already have gestational diabetes, following a low-GI diet can reduce the odds of needing insulin therapy during pregnancy. Additionally, following a low-GI diet may improve your glucose tolerance post-delivery if you had gestational diabetes, and it may aid in weight loss.

Consume an Adequate Number of Servings Per Food Group: That means six or more daily servings of grains, beans, and starchy vegetables; three to five servings of vegetables; two to three servings of fruits; four servings of milk and dairy; and two to three servings of protein (fish, meat, eggs, nuts and beans).

Eat Breakfast: When you first get up in the morning, your body is in a fasting state. It now needs a source of carbohydrates to ensure that your blood sugar does not fall below the norm.

Read Food Labels: This will help you know how many grams of carbohydrates are in a given serving of food so you can calculate how much of a particular food you should eat to get enough carbs without getting too much. When reading a food label, keep in mind that all of the information listed on the nutrition facts panel is for a single serving of that food (see page 164).

Avoid Foods with Added Sugars: This includes sodas, candy, pastries, ice cream, and fruit juice. Avoiding these will also help reduce your risk of excessive weight gain and prevent the consumption of excess calories and sugar.

Go for Optimal Weight Gain: Aim to gain the amount of weight during pregnancy that is recommended for you. To accomplish this, try following the tips outlined in chapter 8.

Consider Following a Mediterranean Diet: A Mediterranean-style diet—which involves high consumption of olive oil, legumes, and fruits and vegetables; moderate consumption of fish and dairy; and low consumption of meat—may be beneficial for controlling your blood sugar, as well as reducing your risk for cardiovascular disease.

Stay Active: Try to get as much physical activity as you can; regular exercise will help regulate your blood sugar levels because it uses glucose to provide energy to your body's cells. Aim for at least 30 minutes of physical activity per day—and this doesn't have to be half an hour of gym time. Moderate-intensity activities, such as brisk walking, yoga, Pilates, biking, swimming, or jogging, are all great options. If you can't dedicate a half an hour at a time for physical activity, doing several shorter workouts (for example, three 10-minute periods) throughout the day can be just as beneficial and will help control your blood sugar levels.

Eat Your Fiber: Consume at least the recommended amount of 28 g of fiber per day.

Eat Your Fish: Increase your intake of foods containing omega-3 fatty acids (EPA and DHA) from fatty fish. In fact, try to eat fish, particularly fatty fish, at least two times per week (up to 12 ounces per week).

Eat Your Whole Grains: Consume at least half of all grains as whole grains.

Limit Your Salt: Limit your sodium intake to 2.3 g/day (if you have both gestational diabetes and hypertension, you may need to reduce your sodium intake even further).

ARE YOU GETTING ENOUGH VITAMIN D?

Current research suggests a link between low vitamin D status during pregnancy and abnormal processing of glucose (insulin resistance), and data shows that women who develop gestational diabetes are more likely to be vitamin D deficient. In fact, the majority of our population is vitamin D insufficient or deficient. It is therefore a good idea to get your vitamin D levels checked out (if you haven't done so already) and make sure you are consuming enough vitamin D in your diet. You need at least 15 mcg of vitamin D per day during pregnancy; again, good sources are fortified milk, orange juice, and cereal, as well as fatty fish (such as salmon, catfish, and sardines) and eggs (vitamin D is only in the yolk, however). If you're struggling to meet the requirement, or you want to make sure that you're getting enough on a daily basis, consider taking a supplement. Though science hasn't proved that vitamin D supplementation helps to reduce the risk of developing gestational diabetes, several studies are currently under way to investigate this possibility. However, remember that vitamin D is beneficial for a plethora of other things, such as healthy bone and brain development of your baby, so getting adequate levels is undoubtedly important.

You're Having Twins

Being pregnant with twins can be a real blessing—you are awaiting the arrival of two beautiful babies, both at the same time! However, carrying twins also means greater risk of some pregnancy complications, including increased risk of high blood pressure, preeclampsia, Cesarean delivery, abnormal bleeding, placental abruption, postpartum hemorrhage, iron-deficiency anemia, and others. Two of the biggest concerns for your baby are premature delivery and low birth weight, which makes optimal nutrition and optimal weight gain absolutely essential. That said, don't be too alarmed; you will be getting extra attention from your doctor and will be regularly monitored to ensure that you and your two little ones are happy and healthy throughout your pregnancy. To make sure that your babies are born at or as close to term as possible and with better health outcomes, you should follow the general prenatal nutrition recommendations regarding a balanced diet, as well as gain an appropriate amount of weight. In addition, you'll need to take a few extra steps to ensure that you get all the nutrients you need, because your requirements are much higher than they would be with a singleton pregnancy. This section contains a summary of the tips for a twin pregnancy, with recommendations for weight gain, caloric intake, and nutrient supplementation.

- **Optimal weight gain.** First and most important, you will need to gain quite a few more pounds than the weight gain needed in a singleton pregnancy. As is true for women pregnant with a single baby, weight gain guidelines for women expecting twins are based on a women's pre-pregnancy BMI. A recent study looking at weight gain patterns in twin pregnancies found good and bad news. First, prepregnancy BMI was not predictive of the amount of weight gained in twin pregnancies, unlike what is often seen in singleton pregnancies. However, this study also found that 46 percent of the women in the study sample gained excessive weight, underscoring the importance of healthy eating and exercise patterns throughout your pregnancy.

- **Weight gain rate.** You should aim to gain an appropriate amount of weight by mid-gestation, as the weight that you gain by 24 weeks of gestation has the greatest impact on your babies' growth and birth weight. Gaining 24 pounds by 24 weeks of gestation has been associated with favorable twin outcomes. A low rate of weight gain by 24 weeks, on the other hand, has been associated with poor growth and early delivery,

what to eat when you're pregnant

even if enough weight was gained after the 24th week. A recent study looking at the weight gain patterns of women carrying twins found that those with inadequate weight gain by weeks 20 through 28 of gestation had twice the risk of preterm birth (birth before 32 weeks). Gaining an adequate amount of weight early on will ensure optimal placental growth as well as improve your nutritional stores, both of which will help provide an adequate supply of nutrients to your little ones later in the pregnancy.

BMI-Specific Dietary Recommendations for Twin Pregnancy

	Underweight (BMI <19)	Normal Weight (BMI 19 to 24)	Overweight (BMI 25 to 29)	Obese (BMI >30)
Calories (kcal)	4,000	3,000 to 3,500	3,250	2,700 to 3,000
Protein (g; 20%)	200	175	163	150
Carbohydrates (g; 40%)	400	350	325	300
Fat (g; 40%)	178	156	144	133

Note: The BMI ranges are different from those used now because the recommendations came out before the reclassification of the BMI ranges.

Source: From Goodnight W and Newman R, "Optimal nutrition for improved twin pregnancy outcome." Obstetrics and Gynecology 2009;114(5):1121-34.

- **Meal frequency.** To get an adequate amount of calories and nutrients, you should aim for three meals and about three snacks per day. This will also help reduce the odds of developing hypoglycemia or low blood sugar during your pregnancy.

- **Increased nutritional requirements.** In addition to gaining more weight than with a singleton pregnancy, your nutritional requirements are different than those of women expecting one baby. Your iron needs, for example, are nearly twice as high as theirs are. You also have increased calcium, vitamin D, magnesium, zinc, folic acid, and vitamins C and E needs. Although no official guidelines have yet been established, the expert recommendation is to take a daily supplement (in addition to a prenatal vitamin) for each of these nutrients. In studies of singleton pregnancies, adequate intake of most of these vitamins and minerals has been associated with decreased risk of premature birth and preeclampsia, as

Twin Pregnancy Nutritional Recommendations for Supplementation

Intervention	First Trimester	Second Trimester	Third Trimester
Caloric requirements per day for normal BMI	40 to 45 calories per kg of body weight per day	Alter as necessary for weight gain goal	Alter as necessary for weight gain goal
Caloric requirements per day for underweight BMI	42 to 50 calories per kg of body weight per day	Alter as necessary for weight gain goal	Alter as necessary for weight gain goal
Caloric requirements per day for overweight/ obese BMI	30 to 35 calories per kg of body weight per day	Alter as necessary for weight gain goal	Alter as necessary for weight gain goal
Iron supplementation in addition to the 27 mg required daily in a singleton pregnancy	One 30 mg tablet per day	Two 30-mg tablets per day	Two 30-mg tablets per day
Calcium (mg/day)	1,500	2,500	2,500
Vitamin D (IU/day)	1,000	1,000	1,000
Magnesium (mg/day)	400	800	800
Zinc (mg/day)	15	30	30
DHA/EPA (mg/day)	300 to 500	300 to 500	300 to 500
Vitamin C (mg/day)	500 to 1,000	500 to 1,000	500 to 1,000
Vitamin E (IU/day)	400	400	400
Folic acid (mg/day)	1	1	1

Source: Adapted from Goodnight W and Newman R, Optimal nutrition for improved twin pregnancy outcome. Obstetrics and Gynecology 2009;114(5):1121–34.

well as other favorable effects, even though research on the particular effects of their supplementation in twin pregnancies is still lacking. Take a look at the table above for the specific supplement amounts of each nutrient that you need, based on the trimester of pregnancy.

- Iron. The rate of iron-deficiency anemia is 2.4 to 4 times higher in twins than in singleton pregnancies. Therefore, iron supplementation (60 to 120 mg of elemental iron) during the first and second trimesters can be beneficial in reducing the risk of preterm delivery and low birth weight, especially if you are iron-deficient. If you are anemic, supplementing with 30 mg/day of elemental iron is recommended, in addition to regularly consuming iron-rich foods like beef, fortified cereals, spinach, and kale. The sources from which you get your carbohydrates and protein also matter. You should focus on low- to medium-glycemic-index carbohydrates and aim to get your protein from fish, lean meat, skin-free chicken, eggs, dried beans, peas, and tofu. For information about the recommended proportions of each of the three macronutrients (protein, carbohydrates, and fat) for a twin pregnancy, see the table on page 199.

WHAT ABOUT BREASTFEEDING TWINS?

There are few evidence-based recommendations for specific dietary modifications when breastfeeding twins. However, some suggestions may be helpful: a diet similar to the one you followed during pregnancy (20 percent of calories from protein, 40 percent from carbohydrate, and 40 percent from fat) is recommended, as well as an extra 1,200 to 1,500 calories per day to ensure adequate milk production (by the second month, you may be producing about 1.2 to 2 liters of milk each day!), and continue to take a prenatal vitamin, including DHA.

References

Chapter 1

Bayol SA, Farrington SJ, Stickland NC. "A maternal 'junk food' diet in pregnancy and lactation promotes an exacerbated taste for 'junk food' and a greater propensity for obesity in rat offspring." *British Journal of Nutrition* 2007;98(4):843–51.

Bocarsly ME, Barson JR, Hauca JM, Hoebel BG, Leibowitz SF, Avena NM. "Effects of perinatal exposure to palatable diets on body weight and sensitivity to drugs of abuse in rats." *Physiology & Behavior* 2012;107(4):568–75.

Carroll RT. *The Skeptic's Dictionary: A Collection of Strange Beliefs, Amusing Deceptions, and Dangerous Delusions.* Hoboken, NJ: Wiley, 2003. Available online: www.skepdic.com.

Chuang CH, Stengel MR, Hwang SW, Velott D, Kjerulff KH, Kraschnewski JL. "Behaviours of overweight and obese women during pregnancy who achieve and exceed recommended gestational weight gain." *Obesity Research & Clinical Practice* 2014;8(6):e577–83.

Epstein RH. *Get Me Out: A History of Childbirth from the Garden of Eden to the Sperm Bank.* New York: Norton, 2011.

Flegal KM, Carroll MD, Kit BK, Ogden CL. "Prevalence of obesity and trends in the distribution of body mass index among US adults, 1999-2010." *Journal of the American Medical Association* 2012;307(5):491–7.

Gross H, Pattison H. *Sanctioning Pregnancy: A Psychological Perspective on the Paradoxes and Culture of Research.* New York: Taylor & Francis, 2007.

Institute of Medicine and National Research Council Committee to Reexamine IOM Pregnancy Guidelines; Rasmussen KM, Yaktine AL, editors. *Weight Gain During Pregnancy: Reexamining the Guidelines.* Washington, DC: The National Academies Press, 2009.

Olson CM, Strawderman MS. "Modifiable behavioral factors in a biopsychosocial model predict inadequate and excessive gestational weight gain." *Journal of the American Dietetic Association* 2003;103(1):48–54.

Rooney K, Ozanne SE. "Maternal over-nutrition and offspring obesity predisposition: Targets for preventative interventions." *International Journal of Obesity* (Lond) 2011;35(7):883–90.

Schulz LC. "The Dutch Hunger Winter and the developmental origins of health and disease." *Proceedings of the National Academy of Sciences* 2010;107(39):16757–8.

Chapter 2

American Congress of Obstetrics and Gynecology. ACOG Committee opinion no. 549: "Obesity in pregnancy." *Obstetrics & Gynecology* 2013;121(1):213–17.

American Pregnancy Association. *Postpartum depression fact sheet.* Washington, DC: 2007.

Andrade AM, Greene GW, Melanson KJ. "Eating slowly led to decreases in energy intake within meals in healthy women." *Journal of the American Dietetic Association* 2008;108(7):1186–91.

Bazhan N, Zelena D. "Food-intake regulation during stress by the hypothalamo-pituitary-adrenal axis." *Brain Research Bulletin* 2013;95:46–53.

Bogaerts AF, Devlieger R, Nuyts E, et al. "Anxiety and depressed mood in obese pregnant women: A prospective controlled cohort study." *Obesity Facts* 2013;6(2):152–64.

Boney CM, Verma A, Tucker R, Vohr BR. "Metabolic syndrome in childhood: Association with birth weight, maternal obesity, and gestational diabetes mellitus." *Pediatrics* 2005;115(3):e290–6.

Calvert C, Thomas SL, Ronsmans C, Wagner KS, Adler AJ, Filippi V. "Identifying regional variation in the prevalence of postpartum haemorrhage: A systematic review and meta-analysis." *PloS One* 2012;7(7):e41114.

Cedergren MI. "Maternal morbid obesity and the risk of adverse pregnancy outcome." *Obstetrics & Gynecology* 2004;103(2):219–24.

Centers for Disease Control and Prevention. *National diabetes fact sheet: National estimates and general information on diabetes and prediabetes in the United States.* Atlanta, GA: US Department of Health and Human Services, Centers for Disease Control and Prevention, 2011.

Chen Q, Sjolander A, Langstrom N, et al. "Maternal prepregnancy body mass index and offspring attention deficit hyperactivity disorder: A population-based cohort study using a sibling-comparison design." *International Journal of Epidemiology* 2014;43(1):83–90.

Chesley SC, Annitto JE, Cosgrove RA. "The remote prognosis of eclamptic women." Sixth periodic report. *American Journal of Obstetrics and Gynecology* 1976;124(5):446–59.

Chu SY, Callaghan WM, Kim SY, et al. "Maternal obesity and risk of gestational diabetes mellitus." *Diabetes Care* 2007;30(8):2070–6.

Chung JH, Melsop KA, Gilbert WM, Caughey AB, Walker CK, Main EK. "Increasing pre-pregnancy body mass index is predictive of a progressive escalation in adverse pregnancy outcomes." *The Journal of Maternal-Fetal & Neonatal Medicine* 2012;25(9):1635–9.

Cogswell ME, Scanlon KS, Fein SB, Schieve LA. "Medically advised, mother's personal target, and actual weight gain during pregnancy." *Obstetrics & Gynecology* 1999;94(4):616–22.

Crozier SR, Inskip HM, Godfrey KM, et al. "Weight gain in pregnancy and childhood body composition: Findings from the Southampton Women's Survey." *The American Journal of Clinical Nutrition* 2010;91(6):1745–51.

Fraser A, Tilling K, Macdonald-Wallis C, et al. "Association of maternal weight gain in pregnancy with offspring obesity and metabolic and vascular traits in childhood." *Circulation* 2010;121(23):2557–64.

Fyfe EM, Thompson JM, Anderson NH, Groom KM, McCowan LM. "Maternal obesity and postpartum haemorrhage after vaginal and Caesarean delivery among nulliparous women at term: A retrospective cohort study." *BMC Pregnancy and Childbirth* 2012;12:112.

Guelinckx I, Devlieger R, Bogaerts A, Pauwels S, Vansant G. "The effect of prepregnancy BMI on intention, initiation and duration of breast-feeding." *Public Health Nutrition* 2012;15(5):840–8.

Hammami M, Walters JC, Hockman EM, Koo WW. "Disproportionate alterations in body composition of large for gestational age neonates." *The Journal of Pediatrics* 2001;138(6):817–21.

Harvey E. "Obesity in pregnancy: Deliver sensitive care." *Nursing* 2011;41(10):42–50.

Hauff LE, Leonard SA, Rasmussen KM. "Associations of maternal obesity and psychosocial factors with breastfeeding intention, initiation, and duration." *The American Journal of Clinical Nutrition* 2014;99(3):524–34.

Hilliard AM, Chauhan SP, Zhao Y, Rankins NC. "Effect of obesity on length of labor in nulliparous women." *American Journal of Perinatology* 2012;29(2):127–32.

Institute of Medicine. "Recommendations for weight gain during pregnancy (figure)." www.iom.edu/About-IOM/Making-a-Difference/Kellogg/HealthyPregnancy.aspx. Accessed July 9, 2014.

Institute of Medicine and National Research Council Committee to Reexamine IOM Pregnancy Weight Guidelines; Rasmussen KM, Yaktine AL, editors. *Weight Gain During Pregnancy: Reexamining the Guidelines*. Washington, DC: National Academies Press, 2009.

Jeyabalan A. "Epidemiology of preeclampsia: Impact of obesity." *Nutrition Reviews* 2013;71 Suppl 1:S18–25.

Jolly MC, Sebire NJ, Harris JP, Regan L, Robinson S. "Risk factors for macrosomia and its clinical consequences: A study of 350,311 pregnancies." *European Journal of Obstetrics, Gynecology, and Reproductive Biology* 2003;111(1):9–14.

Juhasz G, Gyamfi C, Gyamfi P, Tocce K, Stone JL. "Effect of body mass index and excessive weight gain on success of vaginal birth after Cesarean delivery." *Obstetrics & Gynecology* 2005;106(4):741–6.

Kabiru W, Raynor BD. "Obstetric outcomes associated with increase in BMI category during pregnancy." *American Journal of Obstetrics and Gynecology* 2004;191(3):928–32.

Kim C, Newton KM, Knopp RH. "Gestational diabetes and the incidence of type 2 diabetes: A systematic review." *Diabetes Care* 2002;25(10):1862–8.

Kokkinos A, le Roux CW, Alexiadou K, et al. "Eating slowly increases the postprandial response of the anorexigenic gut hormones, peptide YY and glucagon-like peptide-1." *The Journal of Clinical Endocrinology and Metabolism* 2010;95(1):333–7.

Lacoursiere DY, Baksh L, Bloebaum L, Varner MW. "Maternal body mass index and self-reported postpartum depressive symptoms." *Maternal and Child Health Journal* 2006;10(4):385–90.

Li HT, Zhou YB, Liu JM. "The impact of Cesarean section on offspring overweight and obesity: A systematic review and meta-analysis." *International Journal of Obesity* 2013;37(7):893–9.

Lyall K, Munger KL, O'Reilly EJ, Santangelo SL, Ascherio A. "Maternal dietary fat intake in association with autism spectrum disorders." *American Journal of Epidemiology* 2013;178(2):209–20.

Metwally M, Ong KJ, Ledger WL, Li TC. "Does high body mass index increase the risk of miscarriage after spontaneous and assisted conception? A meta-analysis of the evidence." *Fertility and Sterility* 2008;90(3):714–26.

Moore Simas TA, Doyle Curiale DK, Hardy J, Jackson S, Zhang Y, Liao X. "Efforts needed to provide Institute of Medicine–recommended guidelines for gestational weight gain." *Obstetrics & Gynecology* 2010;115(4):777–83.

Myles TD, Gooch J, Santolaya J. "Obesity as an independent risk factor for infectious morbidity in patients who undergo Cesarean delivery." *Obstetrics & Gynecology* 2002; 100(5 Pt 1):959–64.

Norman SM, Tuuli MG, Odibo AO, Caughey AB, Roehl KA, Cahill AG. "The effects of obesity on the first stage of labor." *Obstetrics & Gynecology* 2012;120(1):130–5.

O'Brien TE, Ray JG, Chan WS. "Maternal body mass index and the risk of preeclampsia: A systematic overview." *Epidemiology* 2003;14(3):368–74.

Ogden CL, Carroll MD, Kit BK, Flegal KM. "Prevalence of childhood and adult obesity in the United States, 2011–2012." *Journal of the American Medical Association* 2014;311(8):806–14.

Ogden CL, Carroll MD, Kit BK, Flegal KM. "Prevalence of obesity among adults: United States, 2011–2012." NCHS data brief, no. 131, 2013.

Perlow JH, Morgan MA. "Massive maternal obesity and perioperative cesarean morbidity." *American Journal of Obstetrics and Gynecology* 1994;170(2):560–5.

Robertson E, Grace S, Wallington T, Stewart DE. "Antenatal risk factors for postpartum depression: A synthesis of recent literature." *General Hospital Psychiatry* 2004;26(4):289–95.

Robinson HE, O'Connell CM, Joseph KS, McLeod NL. "Maternal outcomes in pregnancies complicated by obesity." *Obstetrics & Gynecology* 2005;106(6):1357–64.

Schack-Nielsen L, Michaelsen KF, Gamborg M, Mortensen EL, Sorensen TI. "Gestational weight gain in relation to offspring body mass index and obesity from infancy through adulthood." *International Journal of Obesity* 2010;34(1):67–74.

Shub A, Huning EY, Campbell KJ, McCarthy EA. "Pregnant women's knowledge of weight, weight gain, complications of obesity and weight management strategies in pregnancy." *BMC Research Notes* 2013;6:278.

Simpson KR, Thorman KE. "Obstetric 'conveniences': elective induction of labor, Cesarean birth on demand, and other potentially unnecessary interventions." *The Journal of Perinatal & Neonatal Nursing* 2005;19(2):134–44.

Sinha R, Jastreboff AM. "Stress as a common risk factor for obesity and addiction." *Biological Psychiatry* 2013;73(9):827–35.

Sullivan EL, Nousen EK, Chamlou KA. "Maternal high-fat diet consumption during the perinatal period programs offspring behavior." *Physiology & Behavior* 2014;123:236–42.

Suren P, Roth C, Bresnahan M, et al. "Association between maternal use of folic acid supplements and risk of autism spectrum disorders in children." *Journal of the American Medical Association* 2013;309(6):570–7.

Utah Department of Health. "Pregnancy weight gain diagram (figure)." www.baby yourbaby.org/images/pregweightdiagram.gif. Accessed July 9, 2014.

Wall PD, Deucy EE, Glantz JC, Pressman EK. "Vertical skin incisions and wound complications in the obese parturient." *Obstetrics & Gynecology* 2003;102(5 Pt 1):952–6.

Weiss JL, Malone FD, Emig D, et al. "Obesity, obstetric complications and Cesarean delivery rate—a population-based screening study." *American Journal of Obstetrics and Gynecology* 2004;190(4):1091–7.

Wispelwey BP, Sheiner E. "Cesarean delivery in obese women: A comprehensive review." *The Journal of Maternal-Fetal & Neonatal Medicine* 2013;26(6):547–51.

Wojcicki JM. "Maternal prepregnancy body mass index and initiation and duration of breastfeeding: A review of the literature." *Journal of Women's Health* 2011;20(3):341–7.

Chapter 3

Carlson SE. "Docosahexaenoic acid supplementation in pregnancy and lactation." *American Journal of Clinical Nutrition* 2009;89(2):678S–84S.

Carlson SE, Colombo J, Gajewski BJ, Gustafson KM, Mundy D, Yeast J, Georgieff MK, Markley LA, Kerling EH, Shaddy DJ. "DHA supplementation and pregnancy outcomes." *American Journal of Clinical Nutrition* 2013;97(4):808–15.

Caulfield LE, Zavaleta N, Shankar AH, Merialdi M. "Potential contribution of maternal zinc supplementation during pregnancy to maternal and child survival." *The American Journal of Clinical Nutrition* 1998;68(2 Suppl):499S–508S.

Chin RK. "Nausea and vomiting of early pregnancy and pregnancy outcome. An epidemiological study." *British Journal of Obstetrics and Gynaecology* 1990;97(3):278.

Christesen HT, Falkenberg T, Lamont RF, Jorgensen JS. "The impact of vitamin D on pregnancy: A systematic review." *Acta Obstetricia et Gynecologica Scandinavica* 2012;91(12):1357–67.

Cole ZA, Gale CR, Javaid MK, Robinson SM, Law C, Boucher BJ, Crozier SR, Godfrey KM, Dennison EM, Cooper C. "Maternal dietary patterns during pregnancy and childhood bone mass: A longitudinal study." *Journal of Bone and Mineral Research* 2009;24(4):663–8.

Courville AB, Harel O, Lammi-Keefe CJ. "Consumption of a DHA-containing functional food during pregnancy is associated with lower infant ponderal index and cord plasma insulin concentration." *British Journal of Nutrition* 2011;106(2):208–12.

Cross NA, Hillman LS, Allen SH, Krause GF, Vieira NE. "Calcium homeostasis and bone metabolism during pregnancy, lactation, and postweaning: A longitudinal study." *The American Journal of Clinical Nutrition* 1995;61(3):514–23.

da Silva VR, Hausman DB, Kauwell GP, Sokolow A, Tackett RL, Rathbun SL, Bailey LB. "Obesity affects short-term folate pharmacokinetics in women of childbearing age." *International Journal of Obesity* (Lond) 2013;37(12):1608–10.

De-Regil LM, Palacios C, Ansary A, Kulier R, Pena-Rosas JP. "Vitamin D supplementation for women during pregnancy." *Cochrane Database Systematic Reviews* 2012;2:CD008873.

Dietary Reference Intakes for Calcium and Vitamin D. Washington, DC: National Academy of Sciences, 2011.

Fidler MC, Davidsson L, Zeder C, Walczyk T, Marti I, Hurrell RF. "Effect of ascorbic acid and particle size on iron absorption from ferric pyrophosphate in adult women." *International Journal of Vitamin and Nutrient Research* 2004;74(4):294–300.

Food and Nutrition Board. *Dietary Reference Intakes (DRIs): Recommended Intakes for Individuals*. Washington, DC: National Academy of Sciences, 2004.

Greenberg JA, Bell SJ, Ausdal WV. "Omega-3 fatty acid supplementation during pregnancy." *Reviews in Obstetrics and Gynecology* 2008;1(4):162–9.

Hacker AN, Fung EB, King JC. "Role of calcium during pregnancy: Maternal and fetal needs." *Nutrition Reviews* 2012;70(7):397–409.

Hendricks KA, Nuno OM, Suarez L, et al. "Effects of hyperinsulinemia and obesity on risk of neural tube defects among Mexican Americans." *Epidemiology* 2001;12:630–5.

Hoffman JR, Falvo MJ. "Protein—which is best?" *Journal of Sports Science and Medicine* 2004;3(3):118–30.

Hollis BW, Johnson D, Hulsey TC, Ebeling M, Wagner CL. "Vitamin D supplementation during pregnancy: Double-blind, randomized clinical trial of safety and effectiveness." *Journal of Bone and Mineral Research* 2011;26(10):2341–57.

Imdad A, Bhutta ZA. "Effects of calcium supplementation during pregnancy on maternal, fetal and birth outcomes." Paediatric and Perinatal Epidemiology 2012;26:138–52.

Imhoff-Kunsch B, Briggs V, Goldenberg T, Ramakrishnan U. "Effect of n-3 long-chain poly-unsaturated fatty acid intake during pregnancy on maternal, infant, and child health outcomes: A systematic review." *Paediatric and Perinatal Epidemiology* 2012;26 Suppl 1:91–107.

Larqué E, Gil-Sánchez A, Prieto-Sánchez MT, Koletzko B. "Omega-3 fatty acids, gestation and pregnancy outcomes." *British Journal of Nutrition* 2012;107 Suppl 2:S77–84.

Larqué E, Krauss-Etschmann S, Campoy C, et al. "Docosahexaenoic acid supply in pregnancy affects placental expression of fatty acid transport proteins." *The American Journal of Clinical Nutrition* 2006;84:853–61.

Ley SH, Hanley AJ, Retnakaran R, Sermer M, Zinman B, O'Connor DL. "Effect of macronutrient intake during the second trimester on glucose metabolism later in pregnancy." *The American Journal of Clinical Nutrition* 2011;94(5):1232–40.

Ly A, Lee H, Chen J, Sie KK, Renlund R, Medline A, Sohn KJ, Croxford R, Thompson LU, Kim YI. "Effect of maternal and postweaning folic acid supplementation on mammary tumor risk in the offspring." *Cancer Research* 2011;71(3):988–97.

Miller JW, Ulrich CM. "Folic acid and cancer—where are we today?" *Lancet* 2013;381(9871):974–6.

Morales E, Romieu I, Guerra S, Ballester F, Rebagliato M, Vioque J, Tardon A, Rodriguez Delhi C, Arranz L, Torrent M, et al. "Maternal vitamin D status in pregnancy and risk of lower respiratory tract infections, wheezing, and asthma in offspring." *Epidemiology* 2012;23(1):64–71.

MRC Vitamin Study Research Group. "Prevention of neural tube defects: Results of the Medical Research Council Vitamin Study." *Lancet* 1991;338(8760):131–7.

Needham LL, Grandjean P, Heinzow B, et al. "Partition of environmental chemicals between maternal and fetal blood and tissues." *Environmental Science & Technology* 2011;45(3):1121–6.

Pena-Rosas JP, De-Regil LM, Dowswell T, Viteri FE. "Daily oral iron supplementation during pregnancy." *The Cochrane Database of Systematic Reviews* 2012;12:CD004736.

"Position of the American Dietetic Association and Dietitians of Canada: Vegetarian diets." *Journal of the American Dietetic Association* 2003;103(6):748–65.

Prentice A. "Micronutrients and the bone mineral content of the mother, fetus and new-born." *Journal of Nutrition* 2003;1693S–9S.

Ray JG, Wyatt PR, Thompson MD, et al. "Vitamin B12 and the risk of neural tube defects in a folic-acid-fortified population." *Epidemiology* 2007;18(3):362–6.

Robledo CA, Yeung E, Mendola P, et al. "Preconception maternal and paternal exposure to persistent organic pollutants and birth size: The LIFE Study." *Environmental Health Perspectives* 2014;123(1):88–94.

Ronnenberg AG, Venners SA, Xu X, et al. "Preconception B-vitamin and homocyste-ine status, conception, and early pregnancy loss." *American Journal of Epidemiology* 2007;166(3):304–12.

Schaafsma G. "The protein digestibility-corrected amino acid score." *Journal of Nutrition* 2000;130(7):1865S–7S.

Sen S, Iyer C, Meydani SN. "Obesity during pregnancy alters maternal oxidant balance and micronutrient status." *Journal of Perinatology* 2014;34(2):105–11.

Shaw GM, Carmichael SL, Yang W, Selvin S, Schaffer DM. "Periconceptional dietary intake of choline and betaine and neural tube defects in offspring." *American Journal of Epidemiology* 2004;160(2):102–9.

Shaw GM, Finnell RH, Blom HJ, et al. "Choline and risk of neural tube defects in a folate-fortified population." *Epidemiology* 2009;20(5):714–9.

Shaw GM, Todoroff K, Schaffer DM, et al. "Periconceptional nutrient intake and risk for neural tube defect-affected pregnancies." *Epidemiology* 1999;10:711–6.

Shaw GM, Velie EM, Schaffer D. "Risk of neural tube defect-affected pregnancies among obese women." *Journal of the American Medical Association* 1996;275:1093–6.

Shrim A, Boskovic R, Maltepe C, Navios Y, Garcia-Bournissen F, Koren G. "Pregnancy outcome following use of large doses of vitamin B6 in the first trimester." *Journal of Obstetrics and Gynaecology* 2006;26(8):749–51.

Simopoulos ATP, Leaf A, Salem N. "Essentiality of and recommended dietary intakes for omega-6 and omega-3 fatty acids." *Annals of Nutrition and Metabolism* 1999;43:127–30.

Skakkebaek NE, Rajpert-De Meyts E, Main KM. "Testicular dysgenesis syndrome: An increasingly common developmental disorder with environmental aspects." *Human Reproduction* 2001;16(5):972–8.

Snyder HE, Kwon TW. *Soybean Utilization*. New York: Van Nostrand Reinhold, 1987.

Suarez L, Hendricks K, Felkner M, et al. "Maternal serum B12 levels and risk for neural tube defects in a Texas-Mexico border population." *Annals of Epidemiology* 2003;13:81–8.

Suren P, Roth C, Bresnahan M, et al. "Association between maternal use of folic acid supplements and risk of autism spectrum disorders in children." *Journal of the American Medical Association* 2013;309(6):570–7.

Swan SH, Liu F, Overstreet JW, Brazil C, Skakkebaek NE. "Semen quality of fertile US males in relation to their mothers' beef consumption during pregnancy." *Human Reproduction* 2007;22(6):1497–502.

Takimoto H, Hayashi F, Kusama K, Kato N, Yoshiike N, Toba M, Ishibashi T, Miyasaka N, Kubota T. "Elevated maternal serum folate in the third trimester and reduced fetal growth: A longitudinal study." *Journal of Nutritional Science and Vitaminology* 2011;57(2):130–7.

Tande DL, Ralph JL, Johnson LK, Scheett AJ, Hoverson BS, Anderson CM. "First trimester dietary intake, biochemical measures, and subsequent gestational hypertension among nulliparous women." *Journal of Midwifery & Women's Health* 2013;58(4):423–30.

Thomas JD, Abou EJ, Dominguez HD. "Prenatal choline supplementation mitigates the adverse effects of prenatal alcohol exposure on development in rats." *Neurotoxicology and Teratology* 2009;31(5):303–11.

Torjusen H, Brantsaeter AL, Haugen M, et al. "Reduced risk of preeclampsia with organic vegetable consumption: Results from the prospective Norwegian Mother and Child Cohort Study." *BMJ Open* 2014;4(9):e006143.

Vafeiadi M, Vrijheid M, Fthenou E, et al. "Persistent organic pollutants exposure during pregnancy, maternal gestational weight gain, and birth outcomes in the mother-child cohort in Crete, Greece (RHEA study)." *Environment International* 2014;64:116–23.

Viljakainen HT, Saarnio E, Hytinantti T, Miettinen M, Surcel H, Makitie O, Andersson S, Laitinen K, Lamberg-Allardt C. "Maternal vitamin D status determines bone variables in the newborn." *Journal of Clinical Endocrinology and Metabolism* 2010;95(4):1749–57.

Wei SQ, Qi HP, Luo ZC, Fraser WD. "Maternal vitamin D status and adverse pregnancy outcomes: A systematic review and meta-analysis." *Journal of Maternal-Fetal and Neonatal Medicine* 2013;26(9):889–99.

Weinberg ED. "Are iron supplements appropriate for iron-replete pregnant women?" *Medical Hypotheses* 2009;73(5):714–5.

Weinert LS, Silveiro SP. "Maternal-fetal impact of vitamin D deficiency: A critical review." *Maternal and Child Health Journal* 2015;19(1):94–101.

Werler MM, Louik C, Shapiro S, et al. "Prepregnant weight in relation to risk of neural tube defects." *Journal of the American Medical Association* 1996;275:1089–92.

Yajnik CS, Deshpande SS, Jackson AA, Refsum H, Rao S, Fisher DJ, Bhat DS, Naik SS, Coyaji KJ, Joglekar CV, et al. "Vitamin B12 and folate concentrations during pregnancy and insulin resistance in the offspring: The Pune Maternal Nutrition Study." *Diabetologia* 2008;51(1):29–38.

Zhang C, Liu S, Solomon CG, Hu FB. "Dietary fiber intake, dietary glycemic load, and the risk for gestational diabetes mellitus." *Diabetes Care* 2006;29(10):2223–30.

Ziaei S, Norrozi M, Faghihzadeh S, Jafarbegloo E. "A randomised placebo-controlled trial to determine the effect of iron supplementation on pregnancy outcome in pregnant women with haemoglobin > 13.2 g/dl." *BJOG: An International Journal of Obstetrics and Gynaecology* 2007;114(6):684–8.

Chapter 4

American Congress of Obstetrics and Gynecology. "ACOG Practice Bulleting Number 52: Nausea and Vomiting of Pregnancy." *Obstetrics and Gynecology* 2004;103:803–13.

The British Nutrition Foundation Task Force. *Nutrition and Development: Short- and Long-Term Consequences for Health.* London: Wiley-Blackwell for the British Nutrition Foundation, 2013.

Can Gurkan O, Arslan H. "Effect of acupressure on nausea and vomiting during pregnancy." *Complementary Therapies in Clinical Practice* 2008;14(1):46–52.

Chan RL, Olshan AF, Savitz DA, et al. "Maternal influences on nausea and vomiting in early pregnancy." *Maternal and Child Health Journal* 2011;15(1):122–7.

Cowan WM. "The development of the brain." *Scientific American* 241(3):113–33.

Dodds L, Fell DB, Joseph KS, Allen VM, Butler B. "Outcomes of pregnancies complicated by hyperemesis gravidarum." *Obstetrics and Gynecology* 2006;107(2 Pt 1):285–92.

Einarson TR, Piwko C, Koren G. "Prevalence of nausea and vomiting of pregnancy in the USA: A meta-analysis." *Journal of Population Therapeutics and Clinical Pharmacology* 2013;20(2):e163–70.

Festin M. "Nausea and vomiting in early pregnancy." *Clinical Evidence* 2014;03:1405.

Gill SK, Maltepe C, Koren G. "The effectiveness of discontinuing iron-containing prenatal multivitamins on reducing the severity of nausea and vomiting of pregnancy." *Journal of Obstetrics and Gynaecology* 2009;29(1):13–16.

Larsen WJ. *Human Embryology* 3rd edition, New York, NY: Churchill Livingstone, Inc., 2001.

Matthews A, Haas DM, O'Mathuna DP, Dowswell T, Doyle M. "Interventions for nausea and vomiting in early pregnancy." *The Cochrane Database of Systematic Reviews* 2014;3:CD007575

Newman V, Fullerton JT, Anderson PO. "Clinical advances in the management of severe nausea and vomiting during pregnancy." *Journal of Obstetric, Gynecologic, and Neonatal Nursing* 1993;22(6):483–90.

Saberi F, Sadat Z, Abedzadeh-Kalahroudi M, Taebi M. "Acupressure and ginger to relieve nausea and vomiting in pregnancy: A randomized study." *Iranian Red Crescent Medical Journal* 2013;15(9):854–61.

Thomson M, Corbin R, Leung L. "Effects of ginger for nausea and vomiting in early pregnancy: A meta-analysis." *Journal of the American Board of Family Medicine* 2014;27(1):115–22.

USDA Agricultural Research Service. *National Nutrient Database for Standard Reference.* The National Agricultural Library, Release 25, Software v.1.4;2014.

Viljoen E, Visser J, Koen N, Musekiwa A. "A systematic review and meta-analysis of the effect and safety of ginger in the treatment of pregnancy-associated nausea and vomiting." *Nutrition Journal* 2014;13(1):20.

Chapter 5

The British Nutrition Foundation Task Force. *Nutrition and Development: Short- and Long-Term Consequences for Health.* London: Wiley-Blackwell for the British Nutrition Foundation, 2013.

Di Renzo GC, Brillo E, Romanelli M, Porcaro G, Capanna F, Kanninen TT, Gerli S, Clerici G. "Potential effects of chocolate on human pregnancy: A randomized controlled trial." *Journal of Maternal-Fetal and Neonatal Medicine* 2012;25(10):1860–7.

Institute of Medicine. *Dietary Reference Intakes: The Essential Guide to Nutrient Requirements.* Washington, DC: National Academies Press, 2006.

Larsen WJ. *Human Embryology* 3rd edition, New York, NY: Churchill Livingstone, Inc., 2001.

USDA Agricultural Research Service. *National Nutrient Database for Standard Reference.* The National Agricultural Library, Release 25, Software v.1.4; 2014.

Chapter 6

The British Nutrition Foundation Task Force. *Nutrition and Development: Short- and Long-Term Consequences for Health.* London: Wiley-Blackwell for the British Nutrition Foundation, 2013.

Gingras JL, Mitchell EA, Grattan KE. "Fetal homologue of infant crying." *Archives of Disease in Childhood—Fetal and Neonatal Edition* 2005;90(5):F415–F8.

Institute of Medicine. *Dietary Reference Intakes: The Essential Guide to Nutrient Requirements.* Washington, DC: National Academies Press, 2006.

Institute of Medicine and National Research Council Committee to Reexamine IOM Pregnancy Weight Guidelines; Rasmussen KM, Yaktine AL, editors. *Weight Gain During Pregnancy: Reexamining the Guidelines.* Washington, DC: National Academies Press, 2009.

Larsen WJ. *Human Embryology* 3rd edition, New York, NY: Churchill Livingstone, Inc., 2001.

Naumann CR, Zelig C, Napolitano PG, Ko CW. "Nausea, vomiting, and heartburn in pregnancy: A prospective look at risk, treatment, and outcome." *Journal of Maternal-Fetal and Neonatal Medicine* 2012;25(8):1488–93.

Reissland N, Francis B, Mason J. "Can healthy fetuses show facial expressions of 'pain' or 'distress'?" *PLoS One* 2013;8(6):e65530.

USDA. "EPA and DHA content of fish species." Original Food Guide Pyramid Patterns and Description of USDA, Analyses, 2005. www.health.gov/dietaryguidelines/dga2005/report/html/table_g2_adda2.htm. Accessed on July 10, 2014.

USDA Agricultural Research Service. *National Nutrient Database for Standard Reference.* The National Agricultural Library, Release 25, Software v.1.4; 2014.

Chapter 7

Asarian L, Geary N. "Modulation of appetite by gonadal steroid hormones." Philosophical Transactions of the Royal Society of London Series B. *Biological Sciences* 2006;361(1471):1251–63.

Augustine RA, Grattan DR. "Induction of central leptin resistance in hyperphagic pseudo-pregnant rats by chronic prolactin infusion." *Endocrinology* 2008;149(3):1049–55.

Augustine RA, Ladyman SR, Grattan DR. "From feeding one to feeding many: Hormone-induced changes in bodyweight homeostasis during pregnancy." *The Journal of Physiology* 2008;586(2):387–97.

Belzer LM, Smulian JC, Lu SE, Tepper BJ. "Food cravings and intake of sweet foods in healthy pregnancy and mild gestational diabetes mellitus. A prospective study." *Appetite* 2010;55(3):609–15.

Braunstein GD. "Endocrine changes in pregnancy." In Melmed S, Polonsky, KS, Larsen, PR, Kronenberg, HM, eds., *Williams Textbook of Endocrinology*, 12th Edition, Philadelphia, PA: Saunders Elsevier, 2011,819–32.

Butera PC. "Estradiol and the control of food intake." *Physiology & Behavior* 2010;99(2):175–80.

Chen H, Simar D, Lambert K, Mercier J, Morris MJ. "Maternal and postnatal overnutrition differentially impact appetite regulators and fuel metabolism." *Endocrinology* 2008;149(11):5348–56.

Graham JE, Mayan M, McCargar LJ, Bell RC, Sweet Moms Team. "Making compromises: A qualitative study of sugar consumption behaviors during pregnancy." *Journal of Nutrition Education and Behavior* 2013;45(6):578–85.

Grattan DR. "The actions of prolactin in the brain during pregnancy and lactation." *Progress in Brain Research* 2001;133:153–71.

Hirschberg AL. "Sex hormones, appetite and eating behaviour in women." *Maturitas* 2012;71(3):248–56.

Hurley KM, Caulfield LE, Sacco LM, Costigan KA, Dipietro JA. "Psychosocial influences in dietary patterns during pregnancy." *Journal of the American Dietetic Association* 2005;105(6):963–6.

Kim C, McEwen LN, Kieffer EC, Herman WH, Piette JD. "Self-efficacy, social support, and associations with physical activity and body mass index among women with histories of gestational diabetes mellitus." *The Diabetes Educator* 2008;34(4):719–28.

Ladyman SR, Augustine RA, Grattan DR. "Hormone interactions regulating energy balance during pregnancy." *Journal of Neuroendocrinology* 2010;22(7):805–17.

Malassine A, Frendo JL, Evain-Brion D. "A comparison of placental development and endocrine functions between the human and mouse model." *Human Reproduction Update* 2003;9(6):531–9.

Santollo J, Eckel LA. "Estradiol decreases the orexigenic effect of neuropeptide Y, but not agouti-related protein, in ovariectomized rats." *Behavioural Brain Research* 2008;191(2):173–7.

Stephens-Davidowitz S. "What do pregnant women want?" *New York Times*, May 18, 2014.

Strauss JF, Martinez F, Kiriakidou M. "Placental steroid hormone synthesis: Unique features and unanswered questions." *Biology of Reproduction* 1996;54(2):303–11.

Titolo D, Cai F, Belsham DD. "Coordinate regulation of neuropeptide Y and agouti-related peptide gene expression by estrogen depends on the ratio of estrogen receptor (ER) alpha to ERbeta in clonal hypothalamic neurons." *Molecular Endocrinology* 2006;20(9):2080–92.

Wade GN, Schneider JE. "Metabolic fuels and reproduction in female mammals." *Neuroscience and Biobehavioral Reviews* 1992;16(2):235–72.

Westbrook C, Creswell JD, Tabibnia G, Julson E, Kober H, Tindle HA. "Mindful attention reduces neural and self-reported cue-induced craving in smokers." *Social, Cognitive and Affective Neuroscience* 2013;8(1):73–84.

Chapter 8

American Congress of Obstetricians and Gynecologists. "Exercise during pregnancy and the postpartum period." ACOG Committee Opinion No. 267. *Obstetrics and Gynecology* 2002;99:171–3.

Barakat R, Perales M, Bacchi M, Coteron J, Refoyo I. "A program of exercise throughout pregnancy. Is it safe to mother and newborn?" *American Journal of Health Promotion* 2014;29(1):2–8.

Bogaerts AF, Devlieger R, Nuyts E, Witters I, Gyselaers W, Van den Bergh BR. "Effects of lifestyle intervention in obese pregnant women on gestational weight gain and mental health: A randomized controlled trial." *International Journal of Obesity* 2013;37(6):814–21.

Claesson IM, Sydsjo G, Brynhildsen J, Cedergren M, Jeppsson A, Nystrom F, Sydsjo A, Josefsson A. "Weight gain restriction for obese pregnant women: A case-control intervention study." *International Journal of Obstetrics and Gynaecology* 2008;115(1):44–50.

Davenport MH, Ruchat SM, Giroux I, Sopper MM, Mottola MF. "Timing of excessive pregnancy-related weight gain and offspring adiposity at birth." *Obstetrics and Gynecology* 2013;122(2 Pt 1):255–61.

Drehmer M, Duncan BB, Kac G, Schmidt MI. "Association of second and third trimester weight gain in pregnancy with maternal and fetal outcomes." *PLoS One* 2013;8(1):e54704.

Durie DE, Thornburg LL, Glantz JC. "Effect of second-trimester and third-trimester rate of gestational weight gain on maternal and neonatal outcomes." *Obstetrics and Gynecology* 2011;118(3):569–75.

Foxcroft KF, Rowlands IJ, Byrne NM, McIntyre HD, Callaway LK. "Exercise in obese pregnant women: The role of social factors, lifestyle and pregnancy symptoms." *BMC Pregnancy and Childbirth* 2011;11:4.

Herring SJ, Oken E, Haines J, Rich-Edwards JW, Rifas-Shiman SL, Kleinman Sc DK, Gillman MW. "Misperceived prepregnancy body weight status predicts excessive gestational weight gain: Findings from a US cohort study." *BMC Pregnancy and Childbirth* 2008;8:54.

Josefson JL, Hoffmann JA, Metzger BE. "Excessive weight gain in women with a normal prepregnancy BMI is associated with increased neonatal adiposity." *Pediatric Obesity* 2013;8(2):e33–6.

Kong KL, Campbell C, Wagner K, Peterson A, Lanningham-Foster L. "Impact of a walking intervention during pregnancy on post-partum weight retention and infant anthropometric outcomes." *Journal of Developmental Origins of Health and Disease* 2014;5(3):259–67.

Louie JC, Brand-Miller JC, Markovic TP, Ross GP, Moses RG. "Glycemic index and pregnancy: A systematic literature review." *Journal of Nutrition and Metabolism* 2010;2010:282464.

Louie JC, Markovic TP, Perera N, Foote D, Petocz P, Ross GP, Brand-Miller JC. "A randomized controlled trial investigating the effects of a low-glycemic index diet on pregnancy outcomes in gestational diabetes mellitus." *Diabetes Care* 2011;34(11):2341–6.

McGowan CA, Walsh JM, Byrne J, Curran S, McAuliffe FM. "The influence of a low glycemic index dietary intervention on maternal dietary intake, glycemic index and gestational weight gain during pregnancy: A randomized controlled trial." *Nutrition Journal* 2013;12(1):140.

Moses RG, Casey SA, Quinn EG, Cleary JM, Tapsell LC, Milosavljevic M, Petocz P, Brand-Miller JC. "Pregnancy and Glycemic Index Outcomes study: Effects of low glycemic index compared with conventional dietary advice on selected pregnancy outcomes." *The American Journal of Clinical Nutrition* 2014;99(3):517–23.

Mottola MF, Giroux I, Gratton R, Hammond JA, Hanley A, Harris S, McManus R, Davenport MH, Sopper MM. "Nutrition and exercise prevent excess weight gain in overweight pregnant women." *Medicine and Science in Sports and Exercise* 2010;42(2):265–72.

Phelan S, Phipps MG, Abrams B, Darroch F, Schaffner A, Wing RR. "Randomized trial of a behavioral intervention to prevent excessive gestational weight gain: The Fit for Delivery Study." *The American Journal of Clinical Nutrition* 2011;93(4):772–9.

Polley BA, Wing RR, Sims CJ. "Randomized controlled trial to prevent excessive weight gain in pregnant women." *International Journal of Obesity and Related Metabolic Disorders* 2002;26(11):1494–502.

"Pregnancy weight gain chart for different BMI categories." http://diabetes-pregnancy.ca/wp-content/uploads/2011/06/Weight-Gain-Lbs.pdf. Accessed July 11, 2014.

Ruchat SM, Davenport MH, Giroux I, Hillier M, Batada A, Sopper MM, Hammond JM, Mottola MF. "Nutrition and exercise reduce excessive weight gain in normal-weight pregnant women." *Medicine and Science in Sports and Exercise* 2012;44(8):1419–26.

Ruiz JR, Perales M, Pelaez M, Lopez C, Lucia A, Barakat R. "Supervised exercise-based intervention to prevent excessive gestational weight gain: A randomized controlled trial." *Mayo Clinic Proceedings* 2013;88(12):1388–97.

Streuling I, Beyerlein A, von Kries R. "Can gestational weight gain be modified by increasing physical activity and diet counseling? A meta-analysis of interventional trials." *The American Journal of Clinical Nutrition* 2010;92(4):678–87.

Stuebe AM, Oken E, Gillman MW. "Associations of diet and physical activity during pregnancy with risk for excessive gestational weight gain." *American Journal of Obstetrics and Gynecology* 2009;201(1):58 e1–8.

Wolff S, Legarth J, Vangsgaard K, Toubro S, Astrup A. "A randomized trial of the effects of dietary counseling on gestational weight gain and glucose metabolism in obese pregnant women." *International Journal of Obesity* 2008;32(3):495–501.

Chapter 9

American Academy of Pediatrics. "Breastfeeding and the use of human milk." *Pediatrics* 2005;115(2):496–506.

Baker JL, Gamborg M, Heitmann BL, Lissner L, Sorensen TI, Rasmussen KM. "Breastfeeding reduces postpartum weight retention." *The American Journal of Clinical Nutrition* 2008;88(6):1543–51.

Centers for Disease Control and Prevention. "Progress in increasing breastfeeding and reducing racial/ethnic differences: United States, 2000–2008 births." *Morbidity and Mortality Weekly Report* 2013;62(05):77–80.

Dewey KG, Heinig MJ, Nommsen LA. "Maternal weight-loss patterns during prolonged lactation." *The American Journal of Clinical Nutrition* 1993;58(2):162–6.

Dujmovic M, Kresic G, Mandic ML, Kenjeric D, Cvijanovic O. "Changes in dietary intake and body weight in lactating and non-lactating women: Prospective study in northern coastal Croatia." *Collegium Antropologicum* 2014;38(1):179–87.

Gonzalez-Campoy JM, St Jeor ST, Castorino K, Ebrahim A, Hurley D, Jovanovic L, Mechanick JI, Petak SM, Yu YH, Harris KA, et al. "Clinical practice guidelines for healthy eating for the prevention and treatment of metabolic and endocrine diseases in adults: Cosponsored by the American Association of Clinical Endocrinologists/the American College of Endocrinology and the Obesity Society." *Endocrine Practice* 2013;19 Suppl 3:1–82.

Haiek LN, Kramer MS, Ciampi A, Tirado R. "Postpartum weight loss and infant feeding." *The Journal of the American Board of Family Practice* 2001;14(2):85–94.

Haugen M, Brantsaeter AL, Winkvist A, Lissner L, Alexander J, Oftedal B, Magnus P, Meltzer HM. "Associations of prepregnancy body mass index and gestational weight gain with pregnancy outcome and postpartum weight retention: A prospective observational cohort study." *BMC Pregnancy and Childbirth* 2014;14(1):201.

Institute of Medicine and National Research Council Committee to Reexamine IOM Pregnancy Weight Guidelines; Rasmussen KM, Yaktine AL, editors. *Weight Gain During Pregnancy: Reexamining the Guidelines.* Washington, DC: National Academies Press, 2009.

Janney CA, Zhang D, Sowers M. "Lactation and weight retention." *The American Journal of Clinical Nutrition* 1997;66(5):1116–24.

Kac G, Benicio MH, Velasquez-Melendez G, Valente JG, Struchiner CJ. "Breastfeeding and postpartum weight retention in a cohort of Brazilian women." *American Journal of Clinical Nutrition* 2004;79(3):487–93.

Kong KL, Campbell C, Wagner K, Peterson A, Lanningham-Foster L. "Impact of a walking intervention during pregnancy on postpartum weight retention and infant anthropometric outcomes." *Journal of Developmental Origins of Health and Disease* 2014;5(3):259–67.

Loprinzi PD, Smit E, Mahoney S. "Physical activity and dietary behavior in US adults and their combined influence on health." *Mayo Clinic Proceedings* 2014;89(2):190–8.

Ma D, Szeto IM, Yu K, Ning Y, Li W, Wang J, Zheng Y, Zhang Y, Wang P. "Association between gestational weight gain according to prepregnancy body mass index and short postpartum weight retention in postpartum women." *Clinical Nutrition* 2014;pii :S0261–5614(14)00118–6.

National Research Council. *Dietary Reference Intakes for Energy, Carbohydrate, Fiber, Fat, Fatty Acids, Cholesterol, Protein, and Amino Acids (Macronutrients)*. Washington, DC: The National Academies Press, 2005.

Ohlin A, Rossner S. "Trends in eating patterns, physical activity and socio-demographic factors in relation to postpartum body weight development." *The British Journal of Nutrition* 1994;71(4):457–70.

Oken E, Taveras EM, Popoola FA, Rich-Edwards JW, Gillman MW. "Television, walking, and diet: Associations with postpartum weight retention." *American Journal of Preventive Medicine* 2007;32(4):305–11.

Olson CM, Strawderman MS, Hinton PS, Pearson TA. "Gestational weight gain and postpartum behaviors associated with weight change from early pregnancy to one year postpartum." *International Journal of Obesity and Related Metabolic Disorders* 2003;27(1):117–27.

Ostbye T, Peterson BL, Krause KM, Swamy GK, Lovelady CA. "Predictors of postpartum weight change among overweight and obese women: Results from the Active Mothers Postpartum study." *Journal of Women's Health* 2012;21(2):215–22.

Pereira MA, Rifas-Shiman SL, Kleinman KP, Rich-Edwards JW, Peterson KE, Gillman MW. "Predictors of change in physical activity during and after pregnancy: Project Viva." *American Journal of Preventive Medicine* 2007;32(4):312–9.

Rossner S, Ohlin A. "Pregnancy as a risk factor for obesity: Lessons from the Stockholm Pregnancy and Weight Development Study." *Obesity Research* 1995;3 Suppl 2:267s–75s.

U.S. Department of Agriculture and U.S. Department of Health and Human Services. *Dietary Guidelines for Americans, 2010*. 7th edition. Washington, DC: U.S. Government Printing Office, 2010.

Appendix A

American Pregnancy Association. "Herbal tea and pregnancy." Pregnancy Wellness. americanpregnancy.org/pregnancyhealth/herbaltea.html. Accessed July 10, 2014.

Brent RL, Christian MS, Diener RM. "Evaluation of the reproductive and developmental risks of caffeine." *Developmental and Reproductive Toxicology* 2011;92(2):152–87.

Centers for Disease Control. "Estimating foodborne illness: An overview." www.cdc.gov/foodborneburden/estimates-overview.html. Accessed July 10, 2014.

Centers for Disease Control. *Listeria (Listeriosis) Prevention*. 2013. www.cdc.gov/listeria/ prevention.html. Accessed July 10, 2014.

Centers for Disease Control. "Multistate outbreak of listeriosis linked to whole cantaloupes from Jensen Farms, Colorado." www.cdc.gov/listeria/outbreaks/cantaloupes-jensen-farms/082712/index.html. Accessed July 10, 2014.

Centers for Disease Control. "Protecting people from deadly Listeria food poisoning." CDC VitalSigns 2013. www.cdc.gov/vitalsigns/listeria/index.html. Accessed April 6, 2014.

DesRoches A, Infante-Rivard C, Paradis L, Paradis J, Haddad E. "Peanut allergy: Is maternal transmission of antigens during pregnancy and breastfeeding a risk factor?" *Journal of Investigational Allergology & Clinical Immunology* 2010;20(4):289–94.

Environmental Protection Agency. "Fish consumption advice, 2014." www.epa.gov/mercury/advisories.htm. Accessed July 10, 2014.

Ernst E. "Herbal medicinal products during pregnancy: Are they safe?" *BJOG: An International Journal of Obstetrics & Gynaecology* 2002;109(3):227–35.

Foodsafety.gov. "Checklist of foods to avoid during pregnancy, 2014." www.foodsafety.gov/poisoning/risk/pregnant/chklist_pregnancy.html. Accessed April 5, 2014.

Frazier AL, Camargo CA, Malspeis S, Willett WC, Young MC. "Prospective study of peripregnancy consumption of peanuts or tree nuts by mothers and the risk of peanut or tree nut allergy in their offspring." *JAMA Pediatrics* 2014;168(2):156–62.

Jahanfar S, Sharifah H. "Effects of restricted caffeine intake by mother on fetal, neonatal and pregnancy outcome." *The Cochrane Database of Systematic Reviews* 2009(2):CD006965.

Janakiraman V. "Listeriosis in pregnancy: Diagnosis, treatment, and prevention." *Reviews in Obstetrics and Gynecology* 2008;1:179–85.

Kesmodel US, Bertrand J, Stovring H, Skarpness B, Denny CH, Mortensen EL. "The effect of different alcohol drinking patterns in early to mid pregnancy on the child's intelligence, attention, and executive function." *BJOG: An International Journal of Obstetrics and Gynaecology* 2012;119(10):1180–90.

Maslova E, Bhattacharya S, Lin SW, Michels KB. "Caffeine consumption during pregnancy and risk of preterm birth: A meta-analysis." *The American Journal of Clinical Nutrition* 2010;92(5):1120–32.

Maslova E, Granstrom C, Hansen S, et al. "Peanut and tree nut consumption during pregnancy and allergic disease in children—should mothers decrease their intake? Longitudinal evidence from the Danish National Birth Cohort." *The Journal of Allergology and Clinical Immunology* 2012;130(3):724–32.

National Resources Defense Council (NRDC). "Consumer guide to mercury in fish, 2014." www.nrdc.org/health/effects/mercury/guide.asp. Accessed July 10, 2014.

Nykjaer C, Alwan NA, Greenwood DC, Simpson NA, Hay AW, White KL, Cade JE. "Maternal alcohol intake prior to and during pregnancy and risk of adverse birth outcomes: Evidence from a British cohort." *Journal of Epidemiology and Community Health* 2014;68(6):542–9.

O'Keeffe LM, Greene RA, Kearney PM. "The effect of moderate gestational alcohol consumption during pregnancy on speech and language outcomes in children: A systematic review." *Systematic Reviews* 2014;3:1.

Okike IO, Lamont RF, Heath PT. "Do we really need to worry about Listeria in newborn infants?" *The Pediatric Infectious Disease Journal* 2013;32(4):405–6.

O'Neil E. "Developmental Timeline of Alcohol-Induced Birth Defects." In *Embryo Project Encyclopedia*. Arizona State University, 2011. embryo.asu.edu/handle/10776/2101. Accessed July 10, 2014.

The Pew Charitable Trusts. "Pregnant women & listeria: CDC data show high rate of infections for expectant moms." Health Initiatives, 2013. www.pewtrusts.org/en/research-and-analysis/reports/20w/04/pregnant-women-listeria-cdc-data-show-high-rate-of-infections-for-expectant-moms. Accessed July 10, 2014.

Appendix B

ACOG Committee Opinion No. 361. "Breastfeeding: maternal and infant aspects." *Obstetrics & Gynecology* 2007;109(2 Pt 1):479–80.

American Academy of Family Physicians. "Breastfeeding (policy statement), 2007." www.aafp.org/online/en/home/policy /policies/b/breastfeedingpolicy.html. Accessed June 9, 2014.

American College of Nurse-Midwives, Division of Women's Health Policy and Leadership. "Position statement: Breastfeeding, 2004." www.midwife.org/siteFiles/position/Breastfeeding_05.pdf. Accessed June 9, 2014.

American Public Health Association. "A call to action on breastfeeding: A fundamental public health issue, 2007." Policy No. 200714. www.apha.org/advocacy/policy/policysearch/default .htm?id=1360. Accessed June 9, 2014.

Arenz S, Ruckerl R, Koletzko B, von Kries R. "Breast-feeding and childhood obesity— a systematic review." *International Journal of Obesity and Related Metabolic Disorders* 2004;28(10):1247–56.

Bachrach VR, Schwarz E, Bachrach LR. "Breastfeeding and the risk of hospitalization for respiratory disease in infancy: A meta-analysis." *Archives of Pediatric and Adolescent Medicine* 2003;157:237–43.

Baker JL, Gamborg M, Heitmann BL, Lissner L, Sørensen TI, Rasmussen KM. "Breastfeeding reduces postpartum weight retention." *The American Journal of Clinical Nutrition* 2008;88(6):1543–51.

Ballard O, Morrow AL. "Human milk composition: Nutrients and bioactive factors." *Pediatric Clinics of North America* 2013;60(1):49–74.

Beauchamp GK, Mennella JA. "Early flavor learning and its impact on later feeding behavior." *Journal of Pediatric Gastroenterology and Nutrition* 2009;48 Suppl 1:S25–30.

Boghossian NS, Yeung EH, Lipsky LM, Poon AK, Albert PS. "Dietary patterns in association with postpartum weight retention." *The American Journal of Clinical Nutrition* 2013;97(6):1338–45.

Cooke LJ, Wardle J, Gibson EL, et al. "Demographic, familial and trait predictors of fruit and vegetable consumption by preschool children." *Public Health Nutrition* 2004;7:295–302

Dunstan JA, Mitoulas LR, Dixon G, Doherty DA, Hartmann PE, Simmer K, Prescott SL. "The effects of fish oil supplementation in pregnancy on breast milk fatty acid composition over the course of lactation: A randomized controlled trial." *Pediatric Research* 2007;62(6):689–94.

Food and Nutrition Board, Standing Committee on the Scientific Evaluation of Dietary Reference Intakes. "Dietary reference intakes for Vitamin D and calcium." Washington, DC: The National Academies Press, 2010.

Forestell CA, Mennella JA. "Food, folklore and flavor preference development." In: Lammi-Keefe C, Couch SC, Philipson E, eds., 55–64. *Handbook of Nutrition and Pregnancy*. Totowa, NJ: Humana Press, 2008.

Galloway AT, Lee Y, Birch LL. "Predictors and consequences of food neophobia and pickiness in young girls." *Journal of the American Dietetic Association* 2003;103:692–8.

Gartner LM, Morton J, Lawrence RA, Naylor AJ, O'Hare D, Schanler RJ, Eidelman AI. "Breastfeeding and the use of human milk." *Pediatrics* 2005;115(2):496–506.

Haastrup MB, Pottegård A, Damkier P. "Alcohol and breastfeeding." *Basic & Clinical Pharmacology & Toxicology* 2014;114(2):168–73.

Ho E, Collantes A, Kapur BM, Moretti M, Koren G. "Alcohol and breast feeding: Calculation of time to zero level in milk." *Neonatology* 2001;80(3):219–22.

Horwood LJ, Darlow BA, Mogridge N. "Breast milk feeding and cognitive ability at 7–8 years." *Archives of Disease in Childhood* Fetal and Neonatal Edition 2001;84(1):F23-F7.

Ip S, Chung M, Raman G, Chew P, Magula N, DeVine D, et al. "Breastfeeding and maternal and infant health outcomes in developed countries: Evidence report/technology assessment no 153." AHRQ Publication No 07-E007. Rockville, MD: Agency for Healthcare Research and Quality, 2007.

James DC, Lessen R. "Position of the American Dietetic Association: Promoting and supporting breastfeeding." *Journal of the American Dietetic Association* 2009;109(11):1926–42.

Jardri R, Pelta J, Maron M, Thomas P, Delion P, Codaccioni X, Goudemand M. "Predictive validation study of the Edinburgh Postnatal Depression Scale in the first week after delivery and risk analysis for postnatal depression." *Journal of Affective Disorders* 2006;93(1-3):169–76.

Klement E, Cohen RV, Boxman J, Joseph A, Reif S. "Breastfeeding and risk of inflammatory bowel disease: A systematic review with meta-analysis." *The American Journal of Clinical Nutrition* 2004;80(5):1342–52.

La Leche League International. *The Womanly Art of Breastfeeding*. New York: Penguin Books, 1995.

Marques RC, Bernardi JV, Dorea JG, de Fatima RMM, Malm O. "Perinatal multiple exposure to neurotoxic (lead, methylmercury, ethylmercury, and aluminum) substances and neurodevelopment at six and 24 months of age." *Environmental Pollution* 2014;187:130–5.

Mortensen EL, Michaelsen KF, Sanders SA, Reinisch JM. "The association between duration of breastfeeding and adult intelligence." *Journal of the American Medical Association* 2002;287(18):2365–71.

National Research Council. *Dietary Reference Intakes for Energy, Carbohydrate, Fiber, Fat, Fatty Acids, Cholesterol, Protein, and Amino Acids (Macronutrients)*. Washington, DC: The National Academies Press, 2005.

Nicklaus S, Boggio V, Chabanet C, et al. "A prospective study of food variety seeking in childhood, adolescence and early adult life." *Appetite* 2005;44:289–97.

Nommsen LA, Lovelady CA, Heinig MJ, Lonnerdal B, Dewey KG. "Determinants of energy, protein, lipid, and lactose concentrations in human milk during the first 12 months of lactation: The DARLING Study." *The American Journal of Clinical Nutrition* 1991;53(2):457–65.

Owen CG, Martin RM, Whincup PH, Smith GD, Cook DG. "Does breastfeeding influence risk of type 2 diabetes in later life? A quantitative analysis of published evidence." *The American Journal of Clinical Nutrition* 2006;84(5):1043–54.

Panel on Micronutrients, Subcommittees on Upper Reference Levels of Nutrients and of Interpretation and Use of Dietary Reference Intakes, and the Standing Committee on the Scientific Evaluation of Dietary Reference Intakes. "Dietary reference intakes for Vitamin A, Vitamin K, arsenic, boron, chromium, copper, iodine, iron, manganese, molybdenum, nickel, silicon, vanadium, and zinc." Washington, DC: The National Academies Press, 2001.

Skinner JD, Carruth BR, Wendy B, et al. "Children's food preferences: A longitudinal analysis." *Journal of the American Dietetic Association* 2002;102:1638–46.

Sullivan SA, Birch LL. "Infant dietary experience and acceptance of solid foods." *Pediatrics* 1994;93:271–77.

Taylor RW, Grant AM, Goulding A, Williams SM. "Early adiposity rebound: Review of papers linking this to subsequent obesity in children and adults." *Current Opinion in Clinical Nutrition and Metabolic Care* 2005;5:607–12.

USDA Agricultural Research Service. *National Nutrient Database for Standard Reference.* The National Agricultural Library, Release 25, Software v.1.4; 2014.

Valentine CJ, Wagner CL. "Nutritional management of the breastfeeding dyad." *Pediatric Clinics of North America* 2013;60(1):261–74.

Appendix C

Alzaim M, Wood RJ. "Vitamin D and gestational diabetes mellitus." *Nutrition Reviews* 2013;71(3):158–67.

American Diabetes Association. "Nutrition recommendations and interventions for diabetes: A position statement of the American Diabetes Association." *Diabetes Care.* 2008;31:S61-S78.

American Diabetes Association. "Standards of medical care in diabetes—2012." *Diabetes Care.* 2000;25 Suppl 1:S11–63.

American Dietetic Association. Diabetes Care and Education Practice Group. "Ready, set, start counting: How to use carbohydrate counting to keep your blood glucose healthy." http://dbcms.s3.amazonaws.com/media/files/73f9af91-b0af-40c2-8f40-659e53061f12/ADA_Carbohydrate%20counting_large%20print_FINAL.pdf. Accessed July 11, 2014.

American Dietetic Association. "Position of the American Dietetic Association and American Society for Nutrition: Obesity, reproduction, and pregnancy outcomes." *Journal of the American Dietetic Association* 2009;109:918–27.

Atkinson FS, Foster-Powell K, Brand-Miller JC. "International tables of glycemic index and glycemic load values: 2008." *Diabetes Care* 2008;31(12):2281–3.

Benjamin TD, Pridijan G. "Update on gestational diabetes." *Obstetrics and Gynecology Clinics* 2010;27(2):255–67.

Bezerra Maia EHMS, Marques Lopes L, Murthi P, da Silva Costa F. "Prevention of preeclampsia." *Journal of Pregnancy* 2012;2012:435090.

Borberg C, Gillmer MD, Brunner EJ, Gunn PJ, Oakley NW, Beard RW. "Obesity in pregnancy: The effect of dietary advice." *Diabetes Care* 1980;3(3):476–81.

Brantsaeter AL, Haugen M, Samuelsen SO, Torjusen H, Trogstad L, Alexander J, Magnus P, Meltzer HM. "A dietary pattern characterized by high intake of vegetables, fruits, and vegetable oils is associated with reduced risk of preeclampsia in nulliparous pregnant Norwegian women." *Journal of Nutrition* 2009;139(6):1162–8.

California Food Guide: Fulfilling the Dietary Guidelines for Americans. Sacramento, CA: California Department of Health Care and California Department of Public Health, 2008.

Cedergren MI. "Maternal morbid obesity and the pregnancy outcome." *Obstetrics and Gynecology* 2004;103:219–24.

Churchill D, Perry IJ, Beevers DG. "Ambulatory blood pressure in pregnancy and fetal growth." *Lancet* 1997;349:7–10.

Clausen T, Slott M, Solvoll K, Drevon CA, Vollset SE, Henriksen T. "High intake of energy, sucrose, and polyunsaturated fatty acids is associated with increased risk of preeclampsia." *American Journal of Obstetrics and Gynecology* 2001;185(2):451–8.

Cunningham FG, Leveno KJ, Bloom SL, et al. "Diabetes." In Cunningham FG, Leveno KL, Bloom SL, et al., eds. *Williams Obstetrics.* 23rd edition. New York: McGraw-Hill, 2010.

Duley L. "Calcium supplementation during pregnancy for preventing hypertensive disorders and related problems." *Cochrane Database of Systematic Reviews* 2010(8):CD001059.

Eckel RH, Jakicic JM, Ard JD, Hubbard VS, de Jesus JM, Lee IM, Lichtenstein AH, Loria CM, Millen BE, Miller NH, et al. "2013 AHA/ACC Guideline on Lifestyle Management to Reduce Cardiovascular Risk: A Report of the American College of Cardiology/American Heart Association Task Force on Practice Guidelines." *Journal of the American College of Cardiology* 2014;63(25_PA):2960–84.

Evert AB, Boucher JL, Cypress M, et al. "Nutrition therapy recommendations for the management of adults with diabetes." *Diabetes Care* 2013;36(11):3821–42.

Flidel-Rimon O, Shinwell ES. "Breastfeeding twins and high multiples." *Archives of Disease in Childhood,* Fetal and Neonatal Edition 2006;91(5):F377–80.

Goodnight W, Newman R. "Optimal nutrition for improved twin pregnancy outcome." *Obstetrics and Gynecology* 2009;114(5):1121–34.

Guelinckx I, Devlieger R, Beckers K, Vansant G. "Maternal obesity: Pregnancy complications, gestational weight gain and nutrition." *Obesity Reviews* 2008;9(2):140–50.

Han S, Crowther CA, Middleton P, Heatley E. "Different types of dietary advice for women with gestational diabetes mellitus." *Cochrane Database of Systematic Reviews* 2013;3:CD009275.

Haugen M, Brantsaeter AL, Trogstad L, Alexander J, Roth C, Magnus P, Meltzer HM. "Vitamin D supplementation and reduced risk of preeclampsia in nulliparous women." *Epidemiology* 2009;20(5):720–6.

Institute of Medicine and National Research Council Committee to Reexamine IOM Pregnancy Guidelines; Rasmussen KM, Yaktine AL, editors. *Weight Gain During Pregnancy: Reexamining the Guidelines*. Washington, DC: The National Academies Press, 2009.

Inzucchi SE, Bergenstal RM, Buse JB, et al. "Management of hyperglycemia in type 2 diabetes: A patient-centered approach. Position statement of the American Diabetes Association (ADA) and the European Association for the Study of Diabetes (EASD)." *Diabetes Care* 2012;35(6):1364–79.

Jackson AA, Bhutta ZA, Lumbiganon P. "Nutrition as a preventative strategy against adverse pregnancy outcomes." *Journal of Nutrition* 2003;133(5 Suppl 2):1589S-91S.

Kaiser LL, Allen L. "Position of the American Dietetic Association: Nutrition and lifestyle for healthy pregnancy outcome." *Journal of the American Dietetic Association* 2002;103:1479–90.

Kametras NA, McAuliffe F, Krampl E, Chambers J, Nicolaides KH. "Maternal cardiac function in twin pregnancy." *Obstetrics and Gynecology* 2003;102:806–15.

Klein K. "Nutritional recommendations for multiple pregnancy." *Journal of the American Dietetic Association* 2005;105:1050–2.

Lantz ME, Chez RA, Rodriguez A, Porter KB. "Maternal weight gain patterns and birth weight outcome in twin gestation." *Obstetrics and Gynecology* 1996;87(4):551–6.

Luke B, Brown MB, Misiunas R, Anderson E, Nugent C, Van De Ven C, Burpee B, Gogliotti S. "Specialized prenatal care and maternal and infant outcomes in twin pregnancy." *American Journal of Obstetrics and Gynecology* 2003;189(4):934–8.

Luke B, Gillespie B, Min SJ, Avni M, Witter FR, O'Sullivan MJ. "Critical periods of maternal weight gain: Effect on twin birth weight." *American Journal of Obstetrics and Gynecology* 1997;177(5):1055–62.

Luke B, Minogue J, Witter FR, Keith LG, Johnson TR. "The ideal twin pregnancy: Patterns of weight gain, discordancy, and length of gestation." *American Journal of Obstetrics and Gynecology* 1993;169(3):588–97.

Nijdam ME, Timmerman MR, Franx A, et al. "Cardiovascular risk factor assessment after preeclampsia in primary care." *BMC Family Practice* 2009;8(10):77.

Park S, Kim MY, Baik SH, Woo JT, Kwon YJ, Daily JW, Park YM, Yang JH, Kim SH. "Gestational diabetes is associated with high energy and saturated fat intakes and with low plasma visfatin and adiponectin levels independent of prepregnancy BMI." *European Journal of Clinical Nutrition* 2013;67(2):196–201.

Pettit KE, Schrimmer D, Alblewi H, Moore TR, Lacoursiere DY, Ramos GA. "The association between second-trimester weight gain and preterm birth in twin pregnancies." *Obstetrics and Gynecology* 2014;123 Suppl 1:2S.

Pettit KE, Schrimmer D, Alblewi H, Moore TR, Lacoursiere DY, Ramos GA. "Rates of gestational weight gain and postpartum weight retention in term twin pregnancies." *Obstetrics and Gynecology* 2014;123 Suppl 1:166S.

Serlin DC, Lash RW. "Diagnosis and management of gestational diabetes mellitus." *American Family Physician* 2009;80(1):57–62.

Shyam S, Arshad F, Abdul Ghani R, Wahab NA, Safii NS, Nisak MY, Chinna K, Kamaruddin NA. "Low glycaemic index diets improve glucose tolerance and body weight in women with previous history of gestational diabetes: A six months randomized trial." *Nutrition Journal* 2013;12:68.

Sibai BM, Lindheimer M, Hauth J, et al. "Risk factors for preeclampsia, abruption of placentae and adverse neonatal outcomes among women with chronic hypertension." *New England Journal of Medicine* 1998;339:667–71.

Thomas A, Duarte-Gardea M. "Preconception and Prenatal Nutrition." In Samour PQ and King K., eds. *Pediatric Nutrition.* 4th edition. Sudbury, MA: Jones & Bartlett Learning, 2012.

U.S. Department of Agriculture and U.S. Department of Health and Human Services. *Dietary Guidelines for Americans, 2010.* 7th edition. Washington, DC: U.S. Government Printing Office, 2010.

Wolff S, Legarth J, Vangsgaard K, Toubro S, Astrup A. "A randomized trial of the effects of dietary counseling on gestational weight gain and glucose metabolism in obese pregnant women." *International Journal of Obesity* 2008;32(3):495–501.

World Health Organization. "WHO recommendations for prevention and treatment of pre-eclampsia and eclampsia." Geneva: World Health Organization, 2011.

Young BC, Wylie BJ. "Effects of twin gestation on maternal morbidity." *Seminal Perinatology* 2012;36(3):162–8.

Zhang C, Liu S, Solomon CG, Hu FB. "Dietary fiber intake, dietary glycemic load, and the risk for gestational diabetes mellitus." *Diabetes Care* 2006;29(10):2223–30.

Metric Conversion Charts

Volume

1 tablespoon	½ fl oz	15mL
2 tablespoons	1 fl oz	30mL
¼ cup	2 fl oz	60mL
⅓ cup	3 fl oz	80mL
½ cup	4 fl oz	120mL
⅔ cup	5 fl oz (¼ pint)	150mL
¾ cup	6 fl oz	180mL
1 cup	8 fl oz (⅓ pint)	240mL
1¼ cups	10 fl oz (½ pint)	300mL
2 cups, 1 pint	16 fl oz (⅔ pint)	480mL
2½ cups	20 fl oz (1 pint)	600mL
1 quart	32 fl oz (1⅔ pints)	1L

Weight

½ ounce		15g
1 ounce		30g
2 ounces		60g
¼ pound		115g
⅓ pound		150g
½ pound		225g
¾ pound		350g
1 pound (16 ounces)		450g

Oven Temperature

Fahrenheit	Celcius / Gas Mark
250°F	120°C / gas mark ½
275°F	135°C / gas mark 1
300°F	150°C / gas mark 2
325°F	160°C / gas mark 3
350°F	175° or 180°C / gas mark 4
375°F	190°C / gas mark 5
400°F	200°C / gas mark 6
425°F	220°C / gas mark 7
450°F	230°C / gas mark 8
475°F	245°C / gas mark 9
500°F	260°C

Length

¼ inch	6 mm
½ inch	1.25 cm
¾ inch	2 cm
1 inch	2.5 cm
6 inches (½ foot)	15 cm
12 inches (1 foot)	30 cm

About the Author

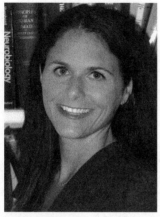

E. Blanchard

Dr. Nicole M. Avena is assistant professor of pharmacology at Mount Sinai School of Medicine; coauthor with John R. Talbott of *Why Diets Fail: Science Explains How to End Cravings, Lose Weight, and Get Healthy*; and an expert in the fields of nutrition, diet, and addiction. She received a PhD in neuroscience and psychology from Princeton University, followed by a postdoctoral fellowship in molecular biology at The Rockefeller University in New York City. Her research has been featured in *Shape, Men's Health, Glamour, Details, Women's Health, Prevention, Oxygen,* and *Fitness,* and she regularly appears on television, including *The Dr. Oz Show, Good Day NY,* and on the Hallmark Channel. She makes public speaking appearances throughout the Unites States, Europe, and Asia. Dr. Avena has written extensively on topics related to food, addiction, obesity, and eating disorders, and she writes the *Food Junkie* blog for *Psychology Today.* She lives with her husband and daughter in New Jersey.

Index

what to eat when you're pregnant

what to eat when you're pregnant